MEDICINE BETWEEN THE LINES

BERNARD LEO REMAKUS, M.D.

221east
Hallstead, PA USA

Medicine Between The Lines
BERNARD LEO REMAKUS, M.D.

Second Edition – October 2014
ISBN:9781499191783

This book is dedicated to my friend,
DR. GEORGE AGURKIS,
who serves as a constant reminder
of all that a man can become
by simply remaining true to
himself, his family and his beliefs.

CONTENTS

BELIEVING EVERYTHING YOU READ

While watching an episode of *Charlie's Angels*, three young ladies, who's IQs were exceeded only by their body temperatures, decided to enroll in detective school. Before they could be admitted to the school, however, they were required to pass an entrance exam.

Upon arriving at the school, each lady was placed in a separate room and briefly shown a mug shot. They were then asked to explain how they would be able to identify the criminal in the future.

"Oh, that's easy," the first lady answered enthusiastically. "The man had only one eye."

"Of course, he had only one eye," the examiner replied sharply. "The mug shot was a profile that showed only one side of his face."

With similar enthusiasm, the second lady answered, "I would be able to identify that man anywhere because he had only one ear."

"Of course, he had only one ear," the examiner shouted. "The photo was a profile and profiles show only one side of a face."

Upon entering the third room, the frustrated examiner decided to give the final candidate some advice. "Take your time and think before answering," he cautioned.

After a prolonged period of thoughtful deliberation, the third lady answered, "I could identify the individual in the photograph by his contact lenses."

Upon confirming from existing records the criminal was wearing contact lenses, the examiner congratulated the young lady. "That's great," he said, "but how were you able to tell the man was wearing contact lenses?"

"Well, I knew he didn't wear glasses," she replied. "With only one eye and one ear, how could he hold the glasses on his face?"

The three young ladies in this story failed their entrance exam because they accepted things at face value. In much the same way, many people fail to understand the real truth behind important issues because they believe everything they read.

By believing everything they read without questioning a writer's credentials, research, conclusions, motivations or affiliations, people unwittingly assimilate a writer's opinions and prejudices and subject themselves to political manipulation. A number of articles recently published in the medical literature clearly demonstrate this point.

The January 5, 2000 edition of the *Journal of the American Medical Association* published a severely flawed research paper that attempted to prove the quality of primary care delivered by nurse practitioners is equal to that of physicians. What the study actually demonstrated was the majority of immigrants who receive free medical care at an American university hospital clinic generally appear satisfied with their care regardless of the professional status of the provider.

Immediately following the publication of this article, newspapers, magazines and internet sites started informing their readers that a prestigious medical journal had reported the quality of primary care delivered by nurse practitioners is equal to that of physicians. As a result, those people who believe everything they read now think nurse practitioners are the professional equivalent of doctors.

This, of course, delights the many managed care executives who now feel free to replace physicians with nurse practitioners, saving megabucks in the process. This, in turn, also delights the many politicians whose political action contributions rise in direct proportion to the increased profitability of the insurance industry.

When people believe everything they read, one misconception can easily set the stage for other misconceptions. *The Harvard Medical Practice Study* is a good example.

Published in 1990, the study called by Ralph Nader, "the best study ever done on medical malpractice," was based on statistics derived from retrospective chart reviews of medical care rendered in a limited number of medical centers (51) in a single state (New York) during a single year (1984). Following wholesale extrapolation and the flagrant omission of multi-site, multi-state and multi-year research data, the study concluded there was more medical malpractice in the United States than was generally acknowledged.

Extrapolation notwithstanding, the Harvard study may have shown there was more medical malpractice in 51 New York medical centers in 1984 than had been previously acknowledged. The study did not and could not prove, however, that what may have happened in New York in 1984 was still happening in the same state and 49 other states 6 years later.

This, of course, did not stop the news media from printing or many readers from believing medical malpractice was some dark secret the medical profession was trying to keep from the American public. Readers were given the opportunity to read about the Harvard study being endorsed by a well-known consumer advocate, but they were never given the opportunity to read about the frequency of frivolous malpractice litigation, physicians winning 85% of court-tried malpractice suits or the paltry 28% of monetary awards victorious plaintiffs were taking home after the legal fees and expenses of malpractice litigation were deducted.

The Harvard study's spurious findings and conclusions, which trial lawyers and legislators quoted freely throughout the 1990s, set the stage for another science fiction classic. This, of course, is the Institute of Medicine's recent report, *"To Err Is Human - Building a Safer Health System."*

In the same spirit of the *Harvard Medical Practice Study*, the Institute of Medicine's report claimed somewhere

3

between 44,000 and 98,000 Americans die yearly because of medical errors. Without questioning how the Institute of Medicine arrived at such numbers or why the range of estimates was so wide, the news media presented the Institute's findings to America's eager readers.

Taking almost as much time as the news media to question the validity or plausibility of the Institute's findings, a number of senators vowed to enact legislation that would curb death by medical error. Millions of taxpayers' dollars from now, the Senate will still be trying to curb a problem that exists only in the wildest extrapolations of a mathematician, but those who believe everything they read will continue to support the Senate's efforts.

A few months ago, another study reported most Americans are happy with their health insurance. Does "most" include the one-million elderly Americans who belong to the 115 health maintenance organizations (HMOs) that plan to abandon their Medicare patients by December 31, 2000 or the millions of Americans who are uninsured or about to become uninsured?

Another study recently reported 83% of the elderly about to be abandoned by their Medicare HMOs live in areas where other HMOs are currently operating. Does the fact many of the "other" HMOs have frozen their enrollments and are not accepting new Medicare patients make one question the true purpose of such studies?

Too many people, including many of our patients and many of our colleagues, believe everything they read. Consequently, the medical profession is currently at the mercy of those who use the medical literature for secondary gain and those who translate the medical literature into laymen's terms and disseminate their own personal translations throughout the news media.

The time has come for more physicians to fight back and help rescue the medical profession from big business, crooked politics and bad press. The time has come for more physicians to publicly display their intellects and expertise and formally challenge the kind of irresponsible research and journalism that is effectively confusing patients and causing them to question the abilities and motivations of the American medical profession.

Every physician has the ability to challenge any medically-related article that appears in print by responding in print. Not only will letters and articles that offer different opinions inject some badly needed intellectual honesty into the medical literature and news media, but they will also convert many who, for lack of an alternative, have no choice but to believe everything they read.

If we have learned anything from the medical literature or news media in recent years, it is that research can be designed to support any pre-existing conclusion. So, don't believe everything you read, especially if the motto of its publisher is "all the news that fits, we print!"

September, 2000

EVIDENCE-BASED MEDICINE

A teenager recently circulated a petition at a high school science fair. The petition called for banning the production of dihydrogen monoxide.

The petition cited the chemical as a potential threat to the global environment and world health. Listed as deleterious effects of dihydrogen monoxide were its capacity to kill or injure if inhaled, promote the formation of acid rain if released into the atmosphere, serve as an environmental hazard at extreme temperatures, act as a solvent for many deadly toxins, and facilitate the growth of both cancer cells and disease-causing microorganisms.

Over 90% of the adults who read about the deadly potential of dihydrogen monoxide signed the petition. In doing so, they unwittingly called for banning the production of water.

Just as these individuals demonstrated an inability to read between the lines of a petition, many physicians are having trouble fully understanding the gist of evidence-based medicine. This research paradigm has been described as the explicit and judicious use of current best evidence from quantitative research in making decisions about individual patients.

In theory, evidence-based medicine is an attempt to have all physicians employing treatment protocols that, through research and statistical analysis, appear to be the best therapeutic options available. In reality, though, the system is a thinly-veiled attempt to have the entire medical profession singing in perfect harmony and practicing medicine from the same cook book.

The major shortcoming of evidence-based medicine is its rejection of medicine as an art. The system's major danger is its potential to be used by outside forces to control the entire medical decision-making process.

Under the false pretense of compliance with evidence-based medicine, government and health insurers could potentially mandate which drugs physicians prescribed, when diagnostic or therapeutic procedures could be obtained and how often patients could see their physicians. Those who control medicine's purse strings could easily sponsor and contrive research studies that resulted in predetermined conclusions.

Under a system of mandatory evidence-based medicine compliance, physicians might not be allowed to prescribe antibiotics unless a patient met all 5 criteria for a bacterial infection, patients might not be allowed to receive more than 2 joint injections yearly and office visits for non-acute illnesses might not be allowed more frequently than every 3 months. These are just a few examples of what might happen if physicians were forced to practice medicine by strict evidence-based medicine protocols.

Under the right conditions, evidence-based medicine could serve as a useful research tool for many physicians. Under other conditions, it could serve as a more useful tool for those bent on socializing American medicine.

As physicians, we must critically analyze research findings and determine if the evidence we are being presented is real or spurious. If we fail to perform this important exegesis, our patients, practices and profession could all wind up in hot dihydrogen monoxide.

May, 2001

STIMULATING THE ECONOMY

I had another one of those crazy dreams again last night. I was spending my first day on the job as Surgeon General and, as I sat at my desk selecting a secretarial pool from a *Victoria's Secret* catalogue, President George W. Bush walked into my office.

"Good morning, General," he said, as he glanced at the cover of my catalogue. "You've been Surgeon General for almost 30 minutes now, and I'd like to know what you've done to earn your keep."

"Well, Sir," I replied without hesitation," I answered the phone a few times, carefully studied this human resources manual I'm holding and worked out an economic stimulus plan."

"Run your stimulus plan by me," the President said.

"Well, to stimulate the economy," I responded, "we have to encourage spending. To encourage spending, we have to create jobs, increase wages and make goods and services more affordable."

"And how do we do that?" the President inquired.

"National health insurance," I replied.

"National health insurance?" the President asked.

"Sure," I answered. "We give every American comprehensive, tax-funded national health insurance. Without having to pay for their employees' health insurance or medical care through Workmen's Compensation programs, both large companies and small businesses will have the money to create more jobs and increase wages."

"We do need more jobs," the President acknowledged.

"But, that's not all," I continued. "Insofar as the cost of employee health insurance contributes to the final price of any manufactured item or provided service, some of the savings brought to companies by national health insurance would be passed on to consumers in the form of less expensive goods and services. This would increase everyone's buying power and allow our industries to become more competitive in both domestic and international markets. Not having to pay for employee health benefits would also allow many small businesses to keep their doors open."

"Hmmm," the President mumbled unequivocally.

"And, furthermore," I continued, "national health insurance would also stimulate the economy by bringing millions of uninsured Americans into doctors' offices and clinics. It would increase hospital revenues by finally paying hospitals for all the care they render to the uninsured and indigent, and stop the tragic and unnecessary closing of American hospitals. It would allow the health care industry to identify and eliminate the costly and unnecessary duplication of services by government and private health insurers, Workmen's Compensation boards and Disability bureaus. It would even permit hospitals and clinics currently being run by Veterans' Affairs and other government agencies to be opened to the general public."

"Is that all?" the President asked jokingly.

"No, Sir," I replied. "National health insurance would also lead to the elimination of medical liability premiums from automobile insurance, homeowner's insurance and business liability insurance, thereby making these private insurances much more affordable for Americans. It would also take much of the strain off our court system by eliminating many of the personal injury lawsuits that follow fender benders, slips on icy sidewalks and injuries in restaurants, stores and other business establishments. After all, without medical bills to pay, most Americans would never consider initiating a personal injury lawsuit."

"We do have too many lawsuits in this country," the President agreed.

"Finally," I concluded, "the institution of a well-structured national health insurance program would help dramatically reduce the cost of health care in America. For starters, a national health insurance program would allow medical malpractice claims to be adjudicated through a federal arbitration process, thereby eliminating the need for physicians to obtain expensive malpractice insurance. By not having to pay exorbitant yearly malpractice insurance premiums, physicians could afford to charge less for their services and still earn more. By no longer being expected to defend frivolous malpractice suits in court, physicians could finally stop practicing so much defensive medicine and stop ordering unnecessary diagnostic tests and consultations. This alone would reduce the yearly cost of health care in America by billions of dollars. This kind of malpractice reform and health care reform would serve as a constant stimulus to the economy. Every American would finally have health insurance, and the taxes resulting from increased company profits, higher wages and more jobs would help pay for it all."

"Good work," the President said, as he quietly confiscated my human resources manual. "So, what's next on your agenda?"

"Trying to figure out why the Surgeon General wears a navy uniform," I answered.

As the President saluted and left the office, I suddenly awoke. I've got to stop eating Tex-Mex food before I go to bed!

February, 2002

PROPACANADA

Propacanada is the term I use to describe the purposeful and systematic dissemination of misinformation about the Canadian health care system by individuals and groups whose special interests would be threatened by the institution of a Canadian-style health care system in the United States. From the recent glut of negative publicity the Canadian health care system has received in many of our leading newspapers and medical journals, it would appear *Propacanada* is on a roll.

A recent ad by a self-proclaimed national policy analysis group attempted to convince readers of the *New York Times* that Canada rations its health care and victimizes ".....the poor, the elderly, rural residents and racial minorities." The ad contended that ".....in Quebec, infant mortality rates are three times greater for the Cree Indians and four times greater for the Inuits (Eskimos) than for the white population." The ad further contended that ".....the United States performs twice as many coronary artery bypass operations per capita on elderly patients as Canada does....."

What this same ad failed to mention was that, on a larger scale, the Canadian health care system is clearly doing better than its American counterpart in terms of overall patient mortality, infant mortality and post-operative mortality. The fact an American infant has a 40% greater chance of dying in its first year of life than a Canadian infant is an alarming, as well as revealing, statistic.

What this ad also failed to mention was an inordinately high percentage of the coronary artery bypass surgery performed in the United States is felt to be unnecessary. It can be argued that, when the clinically unwarranted surgery is removed from the equation, the number of coronary artery bypass procedures performed per capita on

13

American elderly more closely approximates the number performed on Canadian elderly.

In a January, 1993, *Medical World News* article, entitled, *Funding For Canadian National Health Care In Doubt*, it was alleged that ".....there is generally a three-year wait for hip replacement in Canada." In a letter to the editor, published in the February, 1993, edition of the same periodical, a physician responded as follows:

".....I have been practicing in Canada for the last 10 years, and, in my busy practice, after a one- to two-week referral, the patients will get a hip replacement in three weeks. Who is paying you to publish such monumentally absurd lies about the Canadian health care system? Definitely not Canadian doctors or patients. And don't give me that nonsense about Canadians crossing the border to seek health care in the U.S. Just check how many Americans cross the border to get medical care in Canada....."

A recent survey of Canadian physicians, commissioned by the *Medical Post* of Canada, leaves one with the distinct impression the physician who wrote this editorial is not the only physician who feels strongly about the Canadian health care system. Of over 3,000 Canadian physicians surveyed, 83% expressed satisfaction with the Canadian health care system and rated their system as either "very good" or "excellent."

Comments made in the survey were in line with the editorial observation the Canadian health care system ".....incorporates private practice, fee-for-service, the freedom of patients to choose their own physician and freedom of physicians to choose their own patients, and minimal paperwork without intrusion of bureaucrats and businessmen, who believe health care is the place to make profits by harassing doctors and by increasing health insurance premiums and the malpractice system....."

Although Canadian physicians freely admit their health care system is far from perfect, they seem to be thriving in a system that spends 3% less of its gross national product on health care than does the United States, 20% less per capita on health care than does the United States, 10% less of each dollar on health care program administration than does the United States and still manages to provide first trimester pre-natal care to 20% more of its pregnant women than does the United States. Although the Canadian health care system may be far from perfect, it appears to be cost-effective, accessible and appreciated by Canadian physicians and patients alike.

As we continue to debate which health care system is best for the United States, it becomes obvious that many aspects of the Canadian health care system could work in the United States while other aspects of the system might be inconsistent with our current needs and socio-economic ideologies. As we pursue health care reform in this country, we must closely evaluate health care systems, such as the one employed by our neighbors to the North, with an extra measure of intellectual honesty.

The time has come for the United States to forego the distinction of being, with South Africa, one of only two developed nations in the entire world without universal access to health care. Canada may not be able to answer all our questions on health care reform but, *Propacanada* notwithstanding, it may be able to answer more questions than we previously realized.

March, 1993

SMALLPOX

The United States is currently entering a dangerous phase of bioterrorism. Having weathered the initial threat of anthrax, we are now entering a period of false security.

With fewer Americans acquiring anthrax, the shock effect of bioterrorism is starting to wane. Too many people are becoming complacent and forgetting the profound disruption that has already been caused by a bioterrorist who decided to mail a few letters.

At this very moment, untold numbers of bioterrorists may be working in large hospitals across the United States. Consider what might happen if they received a signal to furtively release smallpox into the patient care areas of their hospitals.

Within two weeks, doctors, nurses, hospital workers, patients and recent visitors would become ill and start exhibiting the frightening skin manifestations of smallpox. As a national television audience watched in horror and government officials futilely tried to explain why Americans weren't vaccinated sooner, the families and recent contacts of those with smallpox would begin to experience the non-specific prodrome of their developing illness.

Many of these relatives and contacts would be unaware of their imminent fate as they traveled throughout the United States or other countries. By the time they started noticing changes in their skin, their disease would have already been shared with countless others.

Since World War II, smallpox has been acquired in nonendemic areas mainly by doctors, nurses and patients in hospitals. Disease spread to family, friends and infected cadaver handlers was rapid.

Bioterrorists understand how and where to start an epidemic and they understand wars of terrorism are won by systematically disabling infrastructures. The attacks on the World Trade Center and Pentagon taxed such infrastructures as our military, economy, emergency response systems, insurance industry and travel networks, while anthrax has challenged our postal and delivery services, law enforcement agencies and public health systems.

The United States must continue to guard infrastructures that have yet to be penetrated, such as our refineries, power plants and grids, communications networks, food production resources, and health care delivery system. Explosives can destroy refineries and utilities, and chemicals can destroy food, but smallpox is capable of destroying generations of unprotected health care providers.

Clinically, there are 5 types of smallpox. Hemorrhagic and flat smallpox are usually fatal; ordinary smallpox is fatal in 1-50% of cases; modified smallpox, acquired by previously vaccinated individuals with residual immunity, is rarely fatal; and *variola sine eruptione* is nonfatal smallpox acquired by immune individuals.

Smallpox can be prevented, but not cured once acquired. Survival depends on viral strain, clinical appearance and patient age.

In recent years, government officials have claimed the United States had a stockpile of vaccine capable of preventing smallpox in America for an entire decade. Unfortunately, that stockpile is now outdated, and the safety and efficacy of the vaccine are uncertain.

In September, 2000, the Centers for Disease Control (CDC) awarded Acambis a 20-year, $343 million contract to manage its smallpox vaccine stockpile. In November, 2001, Acambis was awarded a new $428 million contract to manufacture 155 million doses of smallpox vaccine in addition to the 54 million doses previously scheduled to be manufactured in 2002.

What this says is, prior to the year 2000, U.S. intelligence knew smallpox, believed to be missing from U.S.S.R. biowarfare facilities, could be in the possession of bioterrorists. What this also says is government officials currently believe the danger of smallpox being released in the United States through bioterrorism is clear and present.

If the new smallpox vaccine proves both safe and effective, the United States will have enough vaccine to immunize our entire nation against smallpox within one year. Unfortunately, the CDC does not plan to release this vaccine before a first case of smallpox is diagnosed.

Arguments to withhold the vaccine include the perceived global eradication of smallpox; potential side effects of the current smallpox vaccine, such as the development of *vaccinia* in immunocompromised patients and death in as many as 1 per 1 million vaccinated; belief the 12-day incubation period of smallpox would permit a mass vaccination program if and when smallpox occurs; and a possible conflict between smallpox vaccine and other vaccines currently under development. These new vaccines use *vaccinia* as a vector, and those previously immunized against smallpox would have antibodies that could render future vaccines made from *vaccinia* vectors ineffective.

In truth, smallpox virus still exists at various research facilities; the incidence of side effects and death related to vaccination could be significantly reduced through careful patient screening; rapid disease spread could prohibit effective post facto mass immunization of our entire nation; smallpox can be induced by inoculation in as little as 7 days (as compared to the 12 day incubation period of communicable smallpox); and *vaccinia* is only one of many vectors that can be used in vaccine production. What's more, smallpox will not return to America as one new case, but as thousands of new cases, and 25-50% of unvaccinated Americans who acquire smallpox would be expected will die.

The CDC has purchased 209 million doses of smallpox vaccine because it knows smallpox still exists and could be spread by bioterrorists. Our failure to plan for the worst-case scenario of a smallpox epidemic and immunize Americans as soon as a safe and effective vaccine becomes available could make the horrors of September 11, 2001 seem pale by comparison.

If the government waits for cases of smallpox to start appearing in the United States before authorizing vaccination, astonishing numbers of Americans, including many health care providers, could already be dying from the disease. Having disabled our health care infrastructure, terrorists could begin waging a new war against a critically ill nation that was unable to care for itself.

Considering the likelihood of ongoing terrorism and potential of smallpox to reach epidemic proportions in an unvaccinated country, withholding smallpox vaccine from Americans at the present time appears to be shortsighted. Our military has been given adequate munitions with which to fight terrorism abroad, and now the medical profession must be given the weapons required to combat terrorism at home.

Prior to the perceived eradication of smallpox, Americans were routinely immunized against the disease and, even in the absence of new cases of smallpox, the U.S. government had no problem justifying its ongoing smallpox immunization program. Serious side-effects and death are the potential risks of any vaccine but such risks must be accepted if effective national immunization against a life-threatening, communicable disease is to be achieved.

When the British destroyed native American tribes by giving them smallpox-infected blankets during the French and Indian War, biological warfare came to America for the first time. As George Santayana warned in his 1905 classic, *The Life of Reason*, "those who cannot remember the past are condemned to repeat it."

January, 2002

SHOCKS AND AFTERSHOCKS

A few months ago, a drug representative came into my office for the first time to discuss his company's antibiotic. Throughout the course of our conversation, he spoke as if he knew my prescribing habits as well as I did myself.

When I confronted him about his presumptuous attitude, he smugly turned on his laptop computer and retrieved a file that contained an accurate analysis of my antibiotic prescribing history. I watched in disbelief as he guided me through the file and reminded me of the macrolide I prescribed most often, the various cephalosporins I use and how I usually treat uncomplicated urinary tract infections.

You'll probably remember the day when his visit took place. It was the day when an unexplained tremor across the United States temporarily froze the needle at the high end of the Richter Scale.

The bad news is the tremor started from a violent eruption that took place in my office. The good news is the drug rep is starting to recover from his posttraumatic stress syndrome, although he still quivers, cries and calls for his mother whenever he hears antibiotics being discussed.

To say I went ballistic when I discovered my privacy was being invaded by a drug company is a gross understatement. What I later discovered did very little to quell my rage.

It seems drug companies are able to obtain physicians' prescribing information from various pharmacies, insurance companies and marketing groups. The latter specialize in buying prescription records from drug retailers and health insurers, compiling data and reselling the information to drug manufacturers.

The prescription profiles of America's physicians are being bought and sold with very little regard for the privacy of physicians' practices or patient confidentiality. Drug companies use this information to improve their own marketing efforts and sales.

In recent years, a number of large drug companies have entered the health insurance business and a number of health insurers have opened their own pharmacies. Knowledge is power and, in this current information age, the ability to acquire and disseminate physician prescribing data has empowered a rapidly expanding and overlapping segment of corporate America.

The United States experienced another seismic anomaly a few weeks ago. That tremor also started in my office when a patient called to inform me of a letter she received from a drug company.

The letter correctly identified her as a patient who was using a frequently prescribed medication. The letter also extolled the virtues of a new drug the company was currently manufacturing and advised the patient to discuss a trial of the medication with her physician.

Although the phone call did not have the same effect as seeing my prescribing history on a stranger's laptop computer, the effect was still unsettling. I'm not a happy camper when insurance companies try to tell me what medications to prescribe for my patients, and I didn't feel like celebrating when I learned a drug company was trying to convince my patient its new medication was better for her condition than the one I had already prescribed.

In many of the same ways drug companies and health insurers obtain information about physicians' prescribing habits, they also obtain information about the various drugs individual patients are using. Tasteful advertising by drug manufacturers and insurance companies is one thing, but trying to influence drug selection by personally contacting patients and expecting them to deliver the sales pitch to their physicians is an entirely different matter.

America's most recent shockwave occurred a few days ago. I'm happy to report the tremor did not start in my office.

The shockwave started when one of my elderly patients, and countless others like her, received a letter from a lawyer. The letter identified my patient as a former user of a medication that had been taken off the market recently because of alleged side-effects.

In simple language, the letter listed each potential side-effect of the recently discontinued drug. In even simpler language, the letter instructed my patient how to join a class action suit against the drug's manufacturer.

I'm not sure if this latest shockwave started at the drug company's headquarters, the stock market or even the homes of the many patients who benefited from the drug and never experienced any of its purported side-effects. I'm not even sure the tremor wasn't diversionary, as occurs when corporations start class action suits against themselves in an attempt to actively control and limit their exposure in product liability cases.

I am sure the same mechanisms allow drug companies and health insurers to gather physicians' prescribing information and patients' medication lists are also available to law firms and anyone else who can afford the data. I am also sure the gathering of such information is an invasion of physicians' privacy, a threat to patient confidentiality and a clear illustration of the ongoing and unabated socialization of medicine in America.

Blame it on Big Brother or the Bossa Nova, but America's erstwhile sacred institutions are being destroyed. High on the list of these institutions is our once cherished doctor-patient relationship.

When a patient consults a physician, privacy and confidentiality are expected. When a patient purchases a medication, the patient does not expect the pharmacy to sell a record of that sale to a marketing group, the marketers to sell a doctor's prescription profile to a drug

23

company or a drug company to load the information into the laptop computers of its sales force.

The doctor-patient relationship is personal, meaningful and, in many ways, even sacred. A doctor's life work and a patient's illnesses deserve more respect than that accorded through wholesale distribution and irresponsible use.

The medical profession is being taken away from physicians and health care is being wrested from patients by big business and the many politicians, who bless, support and protect corporations legislatively. The end result is health care in a goldfish bowl.

The time has come for more physicians to realize what is happening to health care in America and to start the kind of tremors that will restore respect for our profession. Unless physicians can start a shockwave that will reaffirm our presence, importance and resolve, the medical profession will remain vulnerable to the continued intrusions of big business and government - aftershocks that threaten our very foundations.

December, 2000

KISSES AND LOLLIPOPS

In a memorable scene from *The Hunt For Red October*, the President's National Security Advisor, Jeffrey Pelt, confides in Jack Ryan of the CIA.

"I'm a politician," the advisor says, "...and when I'm not kissing babies, I'm stealing their lollipops!"

On June 29th, President Clinton demonstrated the political art of kissing babies and stealing lollipops in front of a national television audience. The occasion was the long-awaited unveiling of the President's latest plan to reform Medicare.

The highlight of Clinton's Medicare reform plan is a prescription drug benefit program that would pay half of the first $2,000 of drug costs yearly for Medicare patients. Drug costs above $2,000 in any year would have to be paid entirely by the beneficiary.

The drug benefit plan would begin in the year 2002, require a $24 monthly premium and involve no deductibles. The estimated 10-year cost of the program would be $118 billion.

In the year 2008, the drug benefit plan would start paying half of the first $5,000 of yearly drug costs. The monthly premium would rise to $44.

Medicare beneficiaries with annual incomes below $11,000 or elderly couples with incomes below $17,000 would receive prescription drug coverage up to the annual limits without having to pay a monthly premium or their share of the drug costs. Partial financial relief would also be available to other low-income Medicare beneficiaries.

Another highlight of the President's plan is the elimination of Medicare co-payments and deductibles for a limited number of diagnostic tests. The preventive screening tests include: mammograms, prostate cancer screenings and diabetes testing.

In return for the drug benefit plan and preventive screenings, Medicare beneficiaries would be expected to pay a new 20% co-payment for all other diagnostic tests, as well as higher deductibles for office visits and other out-patient treatments. Patients who join Medicare health maintenance organizations (HMOs) would be offered slightly lower monthly premiums to help offset these higher co-payments and deductibles.

In addition to the revenues generated by higher co-payments and deductibles, and the money saved by herding larger numbers of elderly patients into Medicare HMOs, the government plans to save an additional $30 billion over 10 years by reducing Medicare payments to physicians and hospitals, and by earmarking a projected $794 billion from federal government surpluses for the Medicare program. This $794 billion comes from the $1.1 trillion in additional surplus money the Clinton administration claims it recently discovered and can potentially recoup over the next 14 years.

Promising to pay for the prescription drugs of the elderly is a sure way to make headlines and win votes. Unfortunately, when something sounds too good to be true, it usually is.

In sum and substance, the President's latest attempt at reforming the Medicare program is little more than political legerdemain. Our chief political officer has offered the elderly and disabled a limited drug benefit plan that is decidedly inferior to the drug benefit plans already being used by more than two-thirds of Medicare beneficiaries.

Promising to pay $1,000 a year for prescription drugs may sound like great shakes to someone whose last trip to a pharmacy occurred circa World War II, but such a paltry sum would scarcely put a dent in the prescription drug bills of many of today's elderly and disabled patients who require medical treatment for multiple chronic illnesses. What relief will a $1,000 federal stipend bring to those chronically-ill patients whose yearly drug bills will exceed $10,000 by the year 2002?

Similarly, promising to provide mammograms, prostate cancer screenings and diabetes testing without charging Medicare co-payments or deductibles may sound like a good deal, but the federal government's cost for such screening will be a mere fraction of the revenue the government will generate by forcing Medicare beneficiaries to start paying 20% co-payments for all other diagnostic tests, as well as significantly higher deductibles for office visits and all other out-patient treatments. The cost of such screening will also be a mere fraction of the money the government will save by dramatically cutting payments to physicians and hospitals, and by forcing the elderly to join Medicare HMOs when the insurance industry is allowed to make traditional Medicare supplement insurance unaffordable to all but those of independent means.

Many Medicare patients who are forced to pay co-payments for diagnostic testing will attempt to delay or avoid such testing just as many patients who are forced to pay higher deductibles will begin visiting their health care providers less frequently. The Clinton administration realizes this incontrovertible fact and plans to save megabucks for the federal government by creating a scenario in which Medicare patients start refusing diagnostic tests and canceling doctors' appointments because of higher out-of-pocket expenses.

In recent weeks, the President has stated the monthly premium for his Medicare drug benefit plan will have to be doubled in 6 years to help curb inflation. He has also stated his drug benefit plan will be made possible by $1.1 trillion in excess federal surplus that should become available within the next 14 years.

What kind of political doubletalk is this? How can anyone predict trillion-dollar surpluses and, at the same time, warn of Medicare premium hikes because of impending inflation?

For the record, government surpluses are liquidated during periods of inflation and not preserved. For another record, a theoretical $1.1 trillion windfall is just that - theoretical!

Our elderly and disabled desperately need immediate help with the cost of prescription drugs and the cost of health care, but the President's latest Medicare reform plan provides neither. For the benefit of a mere fraction of Medicare beneficiaries, the Clinton administration would increase the financial hardship of the vast majority of elderly and disabled patients who rely on the federal government for their health care.

In reality, curing our ailing health care delivery system would be relatively easy, but those who are currently profiting at the expense of patients and health care providers have too much influence on the politicians who make all the rules. Consequently, the greatest health care delivery system in the history of mankind is currently regressing rather than progressing - as evidenced by the President's latest proposal for Medicare reform.

On June 29th, our nation's political leader loudly promised something too good to be true and then quietly mumbled how much that something would cost. He kissed the baby and stole the lollipop.

Instead of soft-spoken reassurances their pain is being felt, the American people need to start hearing harsh tones directed at those who have been allowed to cause the pain for too many years. Then, maybe, the lollipop could be had for the asking.

August, 1999

CERTIFYING TEAM PHYSICIANS

In the United States today, there are an incredible number of athletic teams that compete in many different sports at various amateur and professional levels. Many of these teams have their own physicians.

At any given moment, a surprisingly large number of physicians are spending time away from their primary care or specialty practices and accompanying amateur softball clubs, college basketball squads and professional football teams to athletic competitions all across the nation. To these many dedicated and competent physicians and the teams they represent, the American Medical Society for Sports Medicine has some disheartening news.

At its recent annual meeting, a member reported team physicians may be risking criminal and civil liability by treating members of their own team during out-of-state competitions. His opinion followed a survey of the directors of the nation's fifty state medical boards.

Although none of the forty-three directors who responded to the survey cited legal action taken by their boards against visiting team physicians, eighteen replied their state did not allow team physicians to treat athletes unless the physicians were licensed to practice medicine in their state. Six directors noted their states required out-of-state physicians to apply for a courtesy license before they were allowed to treat athletes.

Sixteen directors responded their states allowed visiting team physicians to treat athletes as consultants to home team physicians. Only six directors acknowledged their states allowed visiting team physicians to treat athletes without restrictions.

On a separate issue, the responding directors differed on the question of allowable treatment. Thirteen directors replied their states did not allow visiting team physicians to dispense medications to athletes.

In a related survey, sixty-three team physicians from thirty states were questioned about their awareness of the legal restrictions placed on visiting team physicians by various states.
Sixty-eight percent of the physicians surveyed reported being licensed in only one state, but seventy percent admitted to traveling with their teams to out-of-state events.

Seventy-one percent of the physicians surveyed claimed that they were unaware of any state laws that prohibited them from treating athletes at out-of-state competitions, and ninety-three percent admitted they routinely dispensed medications to athletes during such events. Fifty-three percent of the team physicians stated they never contacted home team physicians before traveling to out-of-state competitions, and sixty-six percent stated they didn't consider themselves to be a consultant to a home team physician.

Although the prospect of watching a nationally-televised athletic competition and seeing a qualified physician being arrested for practicing medicine without a license seems remote, such a possibility cannot be entirely dismissed. Related improbabilities that must also be considered include the same physician being entered into the National Practitioner Data Bank for practicing without a license, and the same physician later discovering malpractice committed by an unlicensed physician is not covered under most professional liability insurance policies.

The surveys discussed at the recent meeting of the American Medical Society for Sports Medicine have provided many more questions than answers. For example, how do current state laws impact professional trainers (usually non-physician therapists) who accompany teams to out-of-state athletic competitions and engage in activities that can include minor surgery, injections and the dispensing of medications?

What's more, how do current state laws affect visiting doctors who, while functioning as spectators rather than official team physicians, are asked to treat athletes who are injured or become ill during out-of-state competitions? To this end, exactly what constitutes medical treatment in the setting of athletic competition, and what constitutes "Good Samaritan" intervention by a physician?

Considering the athletic teams requiring their own physicians are the same teams that usually compete in different states, the question of a team physician's professional privileges and restrictions from state to state is one that must be answered. With an ever-increasing number of athletic teams competing in different states, and an ever-increasing number of doctors serving as team physicians or visiting spectators who volunteer their professional services on a need basis, the question is one that should be answered immediately.

It would appear the six states that currently provide temporary courtesy licenses to out-of-state team physicians have the best understanding of the problem at hand. Unfortunately, any practical solution to the problem will have to come from a national, rather than state, level.

It would seem an "American Board of Team Physicians" could be created, and certification by that board used as proof of a physician's competence to treat athletes. Certification by such a board could also be used by physicians as a limited license to treat athletes at officially-sanctioned competitions across the nation.

Insofar as such a board would serve more as a physician registry than a credentialing body, board certification could be a relatively simple process. To become certified and licensed as a team physician, a prospective candidate would merely have to produce an unrestricted medical license, certification by an American specialty board and the formal endorsement of the amateur or professional team for which the physician would be providing medical services during out-of-state competitions.

As a part of its formal endorsement, any team using its own physician would have to provide proof the physician had professional liability insurance that extended to out-of-state and emergency medical services. Teams would also be required to sign a formal agreement that specifically outlined the limits of a physician's treatment of athletes during out-of-state competitions, as well as a protocol for transferring the care of severely injured or ill athletes to health care providers at or in close proximity to competition sites.

As awareness of the recent survey results of the American Medical Society for Sports Medicine spreads, it is inevitable some self-serving public servant will use a photo opportunity to enforce a state law that effectively prohibits visiting team physicians from treating athletes. It may occur in a quiet locker room or on the sidelines of a crowded stadium but, given enough time and lack of corrective action, some unfortunate team physician will be arrested for practicing medicine without a license.

Obviously, such a grim scenario can be obviated. This, of course, will require the concerted efforts of those who currently oversee the activities of medicine and team sports in the United States.

Perhaps the time has come for the state medical boards to sit down with the likes of the American Medical Society for Sports Medicine, the American College of Physicians, the National Collegiate Athletic Association and representatives of America's professional athletic leagues to discuss ways to facilitate the delivery of medical treatment to traveling athletes. Plans to create a national certifying board for team physicians could emerge from such a meeting.

In the meantime, this entire matter can be kept in the proper perspective by realizing circuses travel from one

American city to another with their own doctors, foreign ballet companies bring their own physicians to the United States and Armed Forces doctors work on military bases across the nation without being licensed to practice medicine in the states in which their bases are located. With this in mind, state medical boards should be able to figure out some way to allow a competent team physician to wrap an athlete's ankle on more than one side of a state line.

October, 2000

FOOD SAFETY

While on a business trip a few weeks ago, I decided to grab some lunch at a busy roadside diner. Unfortunately, I never got a chance to sample the establishment's cuisine.

As I entered its restroom, the diner's cook - a somewhat nervous and disheveled youngster, stepped away from the urinal, zipped his fly and quickly returned to the kitchen. He left the restroom without washing his hands.

Having just watched the Dustin Hoffman film, *Outbreak*, the night before, a subconscious preoccupation with disease communicability may have forced me to slightly overreact to the occurrence. Nevertheless, I decided to relinquish any and all rights to the diner's blue plate special and find another place to have lunch.

An hour later, I drove by a large shopping center where a number of fast food restaurants were located. Sensing rapidly waning cholesterol levels, I entered one of the restaurants and quickly sought out a ration of burgers and fries.

As I stood at the counter waiting for my food, the restaurant's manager dropped a stack of empty french fries containers. As she retrieved the containers, her hands touched the dirty tile floor.

I watched in disbelief as the young, seemingly intelligent manager proceeded to touch the insides of several of the containers with her hands, return the entire stack of containers to a dispenser on the counter, and start filling the same containers with french fries. Without taking a few seconds to wash her hands, the young lady continued to spread germs by rubbing her hands along the countertop and against her slacks, handling money and distributing food to customers.

While the manager was repeatedly disregarding the tenets of germ theory, a number of teenage food preparers were also ensuring long nights of gastroenteritis for select customers. Taking apart incorrectly built and previously handled sandwiches, placing slices of cheese, tomatoes and onions from these sandwiches on bare work counters and then reusing them for new sandwiches, and failing to wash their hands after repeated contaminations were just a few of the observable faux pas.

Recently, a number of children contracted Hepatitis A from tainted strawberries they received in their school lunches. The incident shocked millions of Americans and made them question food safety in the United States.

To be sure, food safety leaves a lot to be desired in the United States. In fact, food-borne illnesses are so under-reported by Americans the true scope of the problem is not fully appreciated by as many consumers, health care professionals or public officials as need be.

In the United States today, too much of the food we eat is contaminated during production, transportation, distribution, sale and preparation. Such contamination can be secondary to toxins as well as microbes, and can lead to acute gastro-intestinal illnesses as well as a whole host of chronic diseases.

Insofar as food contamination is a microscopic phenomenon, it can go undetected by even the most scrupulous consumer. What's more, the acute and chronic illnesses that result from food contamination cannot always be traced back to the offending food or contaminant.

Therefore, food poisoning can be misrepresented as food allergy or dietary indiscretion. Similarly, chronic disease can be misunderstood as the result of causative factors that do not include the previous ingestion of contaminated food.

To further complicate matters, there is not universal agreement over the role of certain microorganisms in the etiology of gastro-intestinal illnesses. A good example is gastroenteritis caused by the bacteria, *Pseudomonas aeruginosa*.

Although the medical literature describes Shanghai Fever as a form of gastroenteritis that is caused by *Pseudomonas aeruginosa* and characterized by a 2-week course of fever, abdominal cramps and severe diarrhea, not all infectious disease specialists or gastroenterologists agree gastroenteritis can be caused by species of *Pseudomonas*. Such diversity of opinion, along with the diversity of opinion over the role of certain toxins in gastro-intestinal illness, has further obfuscated the cause-and-effect nature of many diseases that follow the consumption of contaminated food.

Compared to the citizens of many impoverished nations, Americans enjoy a comparatively high standard of food safety. Much more can be done in the United States, however, to improve this safety record.

To this end, the Food and Drug Administration needs to address the issue of food safety with greater vigor. Similarly, state and local health departments need to become more active in ensuring the food people purchase in markets as well as restaurants is safe to eat.

The managers of markets and restaurants also need to become more involved in ensuring food safety. This can be easily accomplished by formally teaching employees how germs and other contaminants are spread, how food contamination can lead to serious illness and how food contamination can be prevented.

Finally, consumers need to become more active in the fight for safer food. Illness thought to be related to contaminated food needs to be brought to the immediate attention of the market or restaurant where the food was purchased and unsanitary conditions in facilities where food is sold needs to be brought to the immediate attention of local health departments.

In his classic book of the same title, Victor Lindlahr observed, *You Are What You Eat.* A quarter-century later, his words are still food for thought!

May, 1997

TEENAGE DRIVING

When a patient dies following a long bout with cancer, someone usually remarks the disease was incurable. When a patient dies from the complications of advanced heart disease, someone usually comments the doctors did all they could to help the patient.

Decades of research and untold amounts of money have been invested in discovering cures for two of the leading causes of death among Americans, namely, cancer and heart disease. To be sure, cures for various forms of cancer and certain varieties of heart disease have been found, but Americans continue to die from these maladies.

A disproportionately high percentage of teenage Americans die not from incurable cancer or untreatable heart disease, but from a cause that can be prevented. I speak, of course, of automobile accidents.

According to National Safety Council statistics, 16- and 17- year-old Americans are involved in three times as many automobile crashes as the rest of the population. On a per-mile basis, 16-year-olds crash twenty times more than the average for all drivers.

Teenage crashes usually result in more injuries and deaths than those involving older drivers because teenagers are twice as likely to have other passengers in their cars at the time of the accident. What's more, teenagers usually wear their seat belts less than half the time.

If you're wondering why teenagers are involved in more crashes than older drivers, the American Automobile Association (AAA) Foundation for Traffic Safety may have some of the answers. In a recent report, the foundation reported "teens are over-represented in crashes caused by driving too fast; driver inattention; overcrowding and running off the road; reckless driving; passing with insufficient distance, in a prohibited passing zone or on the right; and colliding with an animal."

It seems intuitive the poor, and often dangerous, driving habits of many teenagers are due to youthful exuberance and inexperience. Unfortunately, exuberance and inexperience are inadequate justification for property destruction, ever-rising insurance costs and loss of life and limb.

Perhaps the time has come for America to reevaluate which age groups belong behind the wheels of our expensive cars. We have already started coaxing physically-impaired senior citizens to turn in their drivers' licenses, and maybe the time has come to start requiring our teenagers to mature a tad before being given access to the open road.

Once upon a time in America, no one would have dared question the right of 16-year-olds to drive. That, however, was in a day and age when there were fewer drivers on the road, slower cars to drive on slower roads, fewer impaired motorists to confront, a different concept of a car's purpose and its driver's responsibility, and a different respect for the law.

Today, too many teenage drivers take to the highways in a manner reminiscent of a Roman chariot race. Their behavior behind the wheel suggests the same need for speed, recklessness and denial of consequence that is exhibited when these kids play their racing games in a video arcade or cheer the multi-vehicle   pile-ups that appear so innocuous on the silver screen.

Unfortunately, real life auto accidents result in much greater morbidity and mortality than the simulations of video games or cinematic slapstick. As a result, real people are injured, real people die and real lives are changed - sometimes tragically.

If it is true 16-year-olds crash twenty times more than the average for all drivers on a per-mile basis, perhaps 16-year-olds shouldn't be driving. Perhaps 16-year-olds should be allowed to take driver education courses but not licensed to drive until they turn 17.

Following the successful completion of a comprehensive driver's education course, 17-year-olds could be granted provisional licenses which allow them to drive only when accompanied by a licensed driver. After one year of satisfactorily driving under the supervision of other licensed drivers, individuals, 18 years of age and older, could then be allowed to drive without restrictions.

It can be argued 17-year-olds would inherit the current crash rates of 16-year-olds if 16-year-old driving was abolished, but such an argument would be spurious. 17-year-olds are generally more mature than 16-year-olds, and properly educated 17-year-old drivers would be less apt to have accidents if their first year of driving was supervised.

It can also be argued many 16-year-olds need to drive to school and work, but such an argument would also be spurious. The vast majority of American school districts provide school buses for their students, and an inordinately high percentage of American teenagers work for no other reason than to pay for their cars, gas and auto insurance.

We tend to forget 16- and 17-year-olds are still children who need to be taught, supervised and encouraged. We tend to forget suspending the driving privileges of youngsters who drive too fast or too recklessly, who refuse to use seat belts or who drive under the influence of drugs or alcohol makes much more sense than hauling wrecked cars to auto grave yards or wrecked bodies to grave yards reserved for human remains.

Despite medicine's noblest efforts, patients continue to die from incurable disease - and this is unfortunate. At the same time, children continue to die in preventable automobile accidents - and this is inexcusable.

May, 1998

41

THE POOR PAY MORE

Within the next twelve hours, five different people with pneumonia are going to visit the emergency department of the same hospital. Each patient will be examined by the same physician, receive the same diagnostic tests and be discharged with the same medications.

Four of these patients will leave the hospital knowing their health insurance will pay for most, if not all, of their medical services. The one patient who is uninsured will leave the hospital wondering how much he will be billed and how he will pay the bill.

Within the next few days, the hospital will bill four different insurers and one patient identical amounts. The hospital will do so realizing it will ultimately receive five different payments for the same services and a number of these payments will be less than one-half the amount originally billed.

Medicare will pay the hospital one amount and Medicaid another, while the private insurer and health maintenance organization will pay different contractually-discounted fees. Including any existing co-payments and deductibles, the hospital will accept as payment-in-full the amounts it is paid by the various government and private insurers even though the payments vary widely and do not equal the actual billed amount.

The hospital will bill other insurers, including Medicaid, for any amounts approved but not paid by Medicare. In states where Medicaid is not required to make supplemental payments for patients with co-existing Medicare and Medicaid eligibility, the hospital will accept the amount reimbursed by Medicare as payment-in-full.

Although the hospital will bill four insurers the same amount for the same services and accept four different reduced payments in the process, it will not follow the same policy for the one uninsured patient. This patient will be billed the same amount as each of the insurers but expected to pay the total amount billed.

The hospital will resort to any means possible to collect 100% of an outstanding debt owed by an uninsured patient. Collection agencies and small claims courts are just a few of the means the hospital will use to force the uninsured to pay a hospital bill.

Although the hospital may be willing to accept $500 of a $1,000 bill from a government or private insurer, it will be reluctant to offer similar consideration to the uninsured patient. Only as a last resort will the hospital be willing to reduce the amount of a cash debt.

It has been estimated the September 11, 2001 tragedy will ultimately lead to the loss of more than one-half million jobs which will translate into the loss of health insurance for even greater numbers of unfortunate Americans. Now is the time to prepare for the inevitable health care these individuals will require.

While it is enacting other emergency legislation, the federal government should also enact long overdue legislation prohibiting health care providers from charging uninsured patients any fees greater than the amounts they customarily accept as payment-in-full from the government or private insurer with the lowest current fee schedule. If a hospital is able to give discounts to Medicaid or a health maintenance organization, it should be required to do the same for the uninsured.

In 1967, David Caplovitz, observed in his book of the same title, *The Poor Pay More*, and it is obvious the uninsured poor have always paid more for health care. Our entire socio-economic structure was dramatically changed by the events of September 11, 2001, however, and, with less financial wherewithal to provide for the poor, newer ways to ensure access to health care must be developed. March, 2002

THE HARVARD MEDICAL PRACTICE STUDY

Called by Ralph Nader, "the best study ever done on medical malpractice," the *Harvard Medical Practice Study* continues to be regarded by many as the authoritative study on malpractice in the United States. Considering that the study was published in 1990 and based on 1984 data, this is significant.

Although never completely challenged by an authoritative exegesis, the *Harvard Medical Practice Study* has had no small impact on the American medical profession. Without considering the study's validity, legislators, lawyers, insurers, consumer advocates and other special interest groupies have widely used the study as a one-way ticket to the promise land of malpractice reform.

If you're bothered by the fact that ten-year old information is still being used to interpret current malpractice trends, so am I. But that's not all that bothers me about the Harvard study.

I'm also bothered by the fact the *Harvard Medical Practice Study's* statistics were derived from retrospective chart reviews of medical care rendered in a limited number of medical centers (51) in a single state (New York) during a single year (1984). What bothers me about this research design is that medical charts cannot always identify patient injury or physician negligence.

The Harvard study failed to substantiate patients were injured and physicians were negligent. Such substantiation would have required in-depth patient and physician interviews, as well as an exhaustive professional review process.

What also bothers me is the Harvard study researchers conveniently disregarded the possibility that what might be true of medical care in New York might not be true of medical care anywhere else in the United States. Practice patterns, norms and outcomes change with geographic location, and the Harvard study failed to account for a veritable multitude of measurable and immeasurable variables.

For instance, medical care in a private hospital is different than medical care in a teaching institution, just as medical care in the inner city is different than medical care in the suburbs. Medical care by an intern is different than medical care by a board-certified specialist, just as the medical care of an otherwise healthy patient with an uncomplicated illness is different than the medical care of a neglected patient with multiple complicated diseases.

Medical care varies between states, between different cities in the same state and between different hospitals in the same city. The Harvard study operated on an anatomic level when a microscopic investigation was required.

I'm also bothered by the fact malpractice trends in 1984 could not be used to interpret malpractice trends in 1990, much less 1995. American medical care has undergone unprecedented change in the past decade and practice patterns from 1984 are of little more than historical interest a decade later.

The *Harvard Medical Practice Study* reviewed old charts, contrived data and then extrapolated the data to account for practice patterns across the United States. The Harvard study effectively extrapolated a body of inconspicuous errors into a collector's edition of widely-held misconceptions and, in doing so, misled those unfamiliar with scientific research and its limitations.

The Harvard study used its extrapolated data to conclude there was more medical malpractice in the United States than had been generally acknowledged. If the Harvard study is correct, then why are over 85% of court-tried malpractice cases won by physicians?

Could it be a trial format is more effective in evaluating medical treatment than retrospective chart reviews? Could it be the written word is limited in its ability to capture the entire truth of any matter?

The Harvard study used the same data to conclude only one of eight malpractice victims actually sues. If this is correct, then why have the vast majority of American physicians been involved in malpractice suits?

Could it be the actual number of malpractice suits in this country is grossly underestimated? Could it be most of these suits are quietly settled out of court?

If the truth must be told, there have already been too many malpractice suits in the United States - and not too few. The number of frivolous malpractice suits in this country greatly exceeds the number of suits with any semblance of merit.

If the truth must be told, an ever-increasing number of Americans are starting to believe physicians go to medical school to study incompetence as a second language. Unfortunately, as long as prestigious institutions continue to lend their names to quasi-scholarly research and as long as Americans continue to allow celebrities and other gurus do their thinking, their understanding of what constitutes professional competence and responsibility will be incomplete.

Medical malpractice is patient injury caused by physician negligence. It is not maloccurrence or any other subtle deviation from a professional norm.

Before researchers can publish an authoritative report on malpractice, they must fully understand the phenomenon and be able to distinguish it from variations on a similar theme. Before consumer advocates can quote such reports, they must realize their responsibility to protect consumers is no greater than their responsibility to ensure fair treatment to providers.

If the researchers who gave us the Harvard study really want to study the phenomenon of medical malpractice, their study must be redesigned. A multi-year national study that analyzes malpractice trends in each state and employs patient and physician interviews would be much more meaningful than the current Harvard study.

If Ralph Nader really wants to protect consumers, he must also develop a new study design. Maybe he can start by investigating why injured plaintiffs who are true victims of medical malpractice only take home 28% of their court awards.

March, 1995

HMOs

I received an interesting phone call this morning. A young woman called and asked if I would be willing to take care of her daughter the next time she had an asthma attack.

When I asked the woman who her regular doctor was, she identified him as "an HMO doctor." She then went on to complain how this physician was never available when her daughter was having one of her frequent bouts of bronchospasm.

I explained to the woman I did not participate in any health maintenance organizations (HMOs), but that didn't seem to concern her. She explained that, when her daughter was having an asthma attack and her physician was unavailable, she was forced to take her daughter to the emergency room of a hospital that participated in her HMO.

She also explained such inconvenient and time-consuming emergency room visits involved a sizeable co-payment. She reasoned that, for the same price as an emergency room co-payment, she could take her daughter to the private physician of her choice.

Over the past few years, I've received a number of similar calls and heard many complaints about HMOs. In most cases, the patient reported being unwittingly enrolled in an HMO by their employer.

Although most of these patients recalled also being offered conventional health insurance by their employers, they felt such alternative coverage was incomplete and its cost was prohibitive. Nevertheless, lured by the promise of comprehensive health care and a choice of physicians, these patients agreed to join the designated HMOs.

Following a few encounters with their HMOs, most of these patients had the same complaints. For starters, many of these patients felt they were being deprived of medical care by the physician of their choice.

Some of these patients complained about having to leave the care of their former physicians to join an HMO. Other patients complained about the insecurity of having to choose a new physician from a list of unknown names.

Most of these patients felt their care was being rationed by their HMO. They felt too many problems were being handled over the phone, rather than in the office, and their HMOs were using physicians' assistants or nurses in many situations that warranted the attention of a physician.

Many of these patients felt they were being deprived of necessary diagnostic testing by their HMOs and, when testing was scheduled, long waiting periods were involved. They also felt many HMOs were dispensing drugs according to formulary rather than patient need.

Interestingly, many of the patients who kept their former physicians when they joined an HMO, complained about changes in their usual care. In many instances, they felt they were no longer receiving the same care that was being given to patients with conventional health insurance or to those who were paying cash.

To be sure, there are many patients and physicians nationwide who are willing to sing the praises of HMOs. Unfortunately, there are also many patients and physicians who can do nothing but condemn pre-paid health care delivery systems.

In a one-year period between 1985 and 1986, over 80,000 patients left HMOs in the greater Philadelphia area and returned to traditional medical care. As the song goes, "40,000 Frenchmen can't be wrong!"

The concept of the HMO is generally misunderstood and much of this misunderstanding is related to the widespread notion HMOs are handing out something for nothing. Many physicians are lured into HMOs by the expectation of being paid monthly capitation fees if patients are seen or not, while many patients are lured into HMOs by the expectation of free medical care.

Unfortunately, many HMO physicians quickly discover the monthly capitation fees of untreated HMO patients do little to cover the cost of treating the many HMO patients who require frequent treatment, immunizations or in-office diagnostic testing. Many HMO patients quickly discover the "free" medical care from their HMO is not free when co-payments must be paid and when medical care must be obtained outside the HMO.

Still, many physicians continue to join HMOs because of the fear of losing patients to other physicians or being censured by insurance companies or hospitals. Many patients continue to join HMOs because of the inability to afford conventional health care, lack of viable alternatives or sheer naiveté.

In the vast majority of cases, HMO physicians treat their patients according to need rather than operating expense or reimbursement. Every so often, however, an HMO physician tries to cut a few corners and save a few bucks.

The stories of missed diagnoses because of the failure of HMO physicians to examine patients in a timely fashion or fatal outcomes because of the failure of HMO physicians to obtain the necessary diagnostic tests are many. Any physician can miss a diagnosis or fail to obtain a necessary test but, somehow, when this occurs in the shadow of an HMO, the malpractice awards begin to soar to previously untested heights.

I have very little doubt HMOs are generally a poor substitute for conventional medical care. I have even less doubt the concept of HMOs will continue to flourish in the United States and many health care reform proposals will be based on an HMO format.

HMOs are big business. When a California HMO can afford to give its chief executive a $3.4 million yearly bonus, business must be awfully good.

HMOs are good for themselves and good for the businesses that save money by not having to purchase conventional health insurance, but how good are HMOs for patients or physicians? To answer this question, just consider the number of patients that could have been treated in a single year for $3.4 million and the number of financially-strapped physicians' offices that could have been saved for a similar amount.

There are many HMOs that have their own chief executives and dole out millions of dollars in yearly bonuses. Bonuses are based on profits, and big bonuses are based on big profits.

Many generations of Americans grew up believing "you get what you pay for." In the case of HMOs, however, someone else may be getting what you pay for.

September, 1994

GAG CLAUSES

This past April, a physician published an editorial in the local newspaper of a small town in Northeastern Pennsylvania. In his editorial, he questioned the advisability of enrolling Medicare patients in health maintenance organizations (HMOs).

Shortly thereafter, he appeared on local television in a public forum on health care reform. Once again, he questioned the advisability of various health care reform measures.

In August, the concerned physician received a letter from a director of a Northeastern Pennsylvania HMO. Sayeth the HMO:

"Dear Doctor: Our HMO is in the process of recertifying your office for continuing participation. After discussion of your office at the July 1994 Medical Quality Management Committee (QMC) meeting, a concern was identified because it appears that you are not supportive of managed care philosophy. The committee is concerned with the fact that you have 'anti' HMO literature available in your office for our members, and that you have used both television and the newspaper to air your complaints and dissatisfaction with our organization. The QMC recommended we request, in writing, documentation from you as to whether you intend to ameliorate your past attitudes and actions, should you wish to continue to participate in physician network of our HMO. Please respond to this request in thirty days. This information is necessary to complete your recertification…"

In an August interview in the same newspaper, the physician related the only "anti" HMO literature in his office was a copy of his April editorial. Regarding his alleged public criticism of the HMO, he stated: "Why would I? I participate in it. I am concerned, as I wrote, about the Medicare HMO, which isn't even in existence yet..."

The physician viewed his letter from the HMO as "...economic retaliation,...an infringement on my constitutional rights and my freedom of speech...(and) a violation of the doctor/patient relationship." To this end, he is reportedly pursuing legal action against the HMO.

In the same newspaper article, the health maintenance organization defended its letter to the doctor by stating a physician should be supportive of the HMO philosophy. Contractually, the HMO maintains: "Each primary care physician applicant shall be supportive of the managed care philosophy and the concept of the HMO. Each primary care physician shall agree not to take any action or make any communication concerning the HMO with his/her HMO members which reasonably could be expected to undermine the HMO's relationship with HMO members and/or with potential HMO members..."

In insurance circles, such a contractual codicil is known as a "gag" clause. It imposes a "gag" order on HMO providers and, in effect, instructs them to keep their personal opinions to themselves.

Gag orders are not new to the insurance industry, but written gag clauses are becoming more prevalent in provider contracts. In their concerted attempt to totally remove physicians from the health care industry's policy-making loop, health insurers are using contractual gag clauses to gain an upper hand on their providers.

The health insurance industry is bent on getting all American physicians to line dance to the same song. Gag clauses prevent physicians from getting out of line or from trying to dance to a different beat.

Once upon a time, physicians were a respected element in American society. Physicians trained hard for many years and, upon finally achieving professional competence, entered the community and were reimbursed equitably for their services.

Times have changed. Today, physicians are expected to train hard, leave their training with $100,000 educational debts and even greater practice-opening expenses, and render competent and compassionate medical services for fees that couldn't lure many candidates from the welfare rolls.

Medicine was once thought to be either an art or a science. Thanks to our health insurance industry, Medicine has been turned into a business - and a sordid one at that.

For too many years, health insurers have successfully used gag orders, phony audits and sanctions to control physicians and influence physicians' practices and billing patterns. Insurers have isolated individual physicians and, through their various scare tactics, have tried to make these physicians feel like criminals who were somehow lucky to still be practicing medicine.

Too many physicians have given in to the health insurers and chosen to be passive followers, rather than active leaders, in the complicated process of health care reform. The end result is our current mess.

The way to health care reform should be led by health care providers and not by businessmen, lawyers or politicians. Health care is more about people than it is about corporate profits, and the sooner everyone comes to this realization, the sooner we can start to achieve true and lasting health care reform.

Physicians need to become more vocal and more involved in the current health care reform debate. As one concerned physician's case illustrates, there are certain risks to stepping out of line and demanding to be heard, but there are even greater risks to remaining silent and being drafted into an ever-growing army of medical automatons.

Businessmen and politicians are taking over the medical profession and too many physicians are letting them. The very thought of it makes me want to gag.

October, 1994

LIMITING FOREIGN
MEDICAL GRADUATES

The September 7, 1995 edition of the *Medical Tribune* featured an article entitled, *Experts Suggest Limiting FMGs.* In sum and substance, the article contends there are already too many physicians in America, and restricting the number of foreign medical graduates (FMGs) who receive medical training in the United States will alleviate the purported physician surplus.

In this article, the author freely quotes a vice-president for medical education at the Association of American Medical Colleges. This VP is apparently concerned this past decade has witnessed a substantial increase in the number of foreign medical graduates who have entered residency programs in the United States, and three-quarters of these foreign medical graduates have remained in the United States to pursue life, liberty and the right to purchase malpractice insurance.

He alleges the United States has a surplus of physicians and, if the oversupply isn't corrected, "…the United States will invest substantial sums of money to educate physicians who are not needed, and some of the young men and women who pursue careers in medicine may find few professional opportunities when they finish their education." Citing a predicted excess of 165,000 specialists in the United States by the year 2000, the VP argues the overall number of residency positions in the U.S. should remain constant but strict limits should be placed on the number of foreign medical graduates who enter U.S. residency programs.

In this article, the author also quotes the chief of workforce analysis and research at the Bureau of Health Professions. Sayeth the chief: "Our health care costs are spiraling…(and) one way to control those costs is by producing fewer physicians."

I don't know what life looks like outside your office window but, from where I sit, I'd say we have too few physicians in the United States rather than too many. If there were too many physicians in the good old U.S. of A., patients wouldn't be waiting weeks to months for a doctor's appointment, physicians wouldn't be chalking up 60 to 80-hour work weeks and nobody would be talking about physician burnout.

If there were too many physicians in the United States, 100 American counties wouldn't be without a physician, and we wouldn't be graduating physician's assistants, nurse practitioners, certified nurse midwives and other physician extenders in record numbers. If there were too many physicians in America, emergency rooms wouldn't have 4-hour waiting times, and urgent care centers and walk-in clinics wouldn't be overflowing with patients.

If there were too many physicians in the United States, physicians could put in normal work days and return home to normal family lives. This doesn't happen for every American physician because there are not too many physicians in America- there are too few.

So, what would we accomplish by limiting the number of foreign medical graduates who undergo residency training in U.S. hospitals? A sizeable number of these foreign medical graduates are American citizens who were forced to obtain their medical education abroad while still other foreign medical graduates are natives of countries that continue to educate American citizens in their medical schools and still maintain strong diplomatic relations with the United States.

And what's the difference if 75% of the foreign medical graduates who are trained in U.S. hospitals choose to practice medicine in the United States? By remaining in the United States, these physicians are using the skills they acquired in America to treat the illnesses of American patients.

As far as the concern about the United States investing substantial sums of money to educate physicians who are not needed, who ever heard of physicians who weren't needed? America needs each and every one of its physicians - a fact that should become painfully obvious over the next decade as an increasing number of American physicians, who are currently being victimized by the malpractice epidemic, managed care and other manifestations of the current health care reform fiasco, take an early retirement or other form of premature exodus from the medical profession.

As far as the concern about young men and women pursuing careers in medicine only to find few professional opportunities when they finish their education, when's the last time anyone saw a physician standing in an unemployment line? As long as there are sick patients, there will always be employment opportunities for competent physicians.

If you don't believe this, just read the classified ads in any medical publication or major city newspaper. Then, if you still have a tough time accepting the fact employment opportunities abound for American physicians, call any physician placement service and ask for a list of the towns, hospitals and private medical practices that are currently paying big bucks to locate physicians.

As far as the concern about spiraling health care costs, who ever heard of lowering the cost of anything by making it harder to find? If there's one sure way to make the cost of health care spiral to greater heights, it's by making health care less available.

Spiraling health care costs could be contained by flooding the marketplace with health care professionals who were willing to work cheap. Health care costs could never be contained by reducing the number of physicians and making their services more difficult to obtain.

In contrast to many of the assertions made in this recent article, limiting the number of foreign medical graduates who are trained in U.S. hospitals would adversely affect the many U.S. residency programs that typically rely on foreign medical graduates to fill their rosters. At the same time, limiting the number of foreign medical graduates would adversely affect the many physician-shortage areas of the United States that typically rely on foreign medical graduates for their health care.

Before anyone starts talking about limiting entry into the American medical profession, they would be wise to consider the many dire consequences of physician undersupply. The last thing a patient experiencing severe chest pain thinks about is someone's notion there are too many physicians in America.

October 1995

JUST DESSERTS

One night, while watching television, an elderly woman decided to have a snack.

"Would you like some ice cream?" she asked her husband.

"Why, yes," he replied. "I'll have some vanilla, but you better write it down because you know how forgetful you are."

"I won't forget," the wife said. "By the way, would you like anything on your ice cream?"

"Why, yes," the husband answered. "I'd like some strawberries- but you better write it down because you might forget."

"I won't forget," the wife replied, as she retreated to the kitchen.

A short while later, the wife returned with a dish of scrambled eggs.

"I knew you'd forget," the husband said.

"Forget what?" the wife asked.

The husband shook his head and replied, "You forgot the bacon!"

For many years, physicians have embarked on careers in rural medicine with the expectation of strawberry sundaes and other sweet things. Unfortunately, too many rural physicians are still waiting for the ice cream truck to arrive.

Instead of ice cream, the practice of rural medical has brought many physicians cold plates of soggy eggs. In many cases, the plates have been small and the eggs haven't been cooked as ordered.

For the past few months, various newspapers have covered the story of young physicians who have recently opened rural medical practices. Unfortunately, the story is not a new one.

Every few years, another newspaper or magazine reports the story of someone who is trying to make some kind of positive impact in a physician-shortage area. The faces change, as do the towns, but the plot remains the same.

The latest members of the Washington think tank have vowed to ameliorate the problems of America's many physician-shortage areas by luring new physicians into such areas with cash incentives and loan-forgiveness programs. They believe this strategy will bring physicians into the 100 U.S. counties that currently have no physicians.

They also believe this tactic will improve the current ratio of one physician for every 1,000 rural residents. Contrast this to the current ratio of 2.25 physicians for every 1,000 urban residents.

What these philosophers of the Potomac fail to realize is very few American physicians are cut out to be country doctors. This is one of the major reasons why the National Health Service Corps has been such a disappointment.

The vast majority of American physicians were born in urban and suburban areas, have very little understanding of rural America and don't really want to live, work and raise a family in isolated and economically strapped parts of the country. The vast majority of American physicians were trained to be part of a sophisticated health care team and don't really want to be the only medical show in a one-horse town.

The vast majority of American physicians don't want to be perpetually on-call at poorly equipped, inadequately-staffed and financially-strained rural hospitals or work long hours in communities where patients are less likely to have health insurance or qualify for Medicaid. They don't want to be reimbursed by Medicare and other third-party payers at rates that are significantly lower than those paid to physicians who work in urban areas.

The vast majority of American physicians don't want to become scapegoats for peer-review organizations or easy targets for malpractice lawyers. They don't want to live in uncertainty and constantly wonder if managed care will come to the country and force them out of business.

There are many positive things that can be said about living and practicing medicine in the country but not every physician is cut out to be a country doctor. Over 200 rural hospitals have closed in the past decade, and not every physician is comfortable working in a isolated community that may be the next to lose its only in-patient facility.

When all is said and done, America will still have its rural areas and these rural areas will still need physicians. The trick is not to lure new physicians into these areas with easy cash and loan-forgiveness.

When the cash is gone and the loans have been forgiven, the vast majority of these physicians will invariably return from whence they came. Instead, the trick is to create an economic milieu that will allow physicians who feel at home in the country to stay put.

This can be done by improving Medicare, Medicaid and other health insurance reimbursement to rural physicians. It can also be done by making it easier for rural residents to take advantage of government-sponsored health insurance programs and providing financial aid to rural hospitals and related health care facilities.

In recent years, untold numbers of physicians and other health care personnel have been forced to leave rural areas for financial reasons. Positive government intervention to preserve our existing rural health care resources makes more sense than engaging in expensive recruitment efforts of questionable long-term merit.

Politicians want to recruit new physicians to work in rural areas where physicians have traditionally had a difficult time surviving financially. It makes more sense to correct the reimbursement problems particular to rural medicine and retain physicians who are already living and working in the country than it does to recruit new physicians who will have come and gone before the ink has dried on their contracts.

Insofar as individuals born and raised in rural communities are more likely to return to their roots after their formal education has been completed than urban residents are to be transplanted to rural areas, federal and state governments should initiate special programs designed to recruit future physicians and other health care professionals from rural areas. In much the same way programs have been developed to give special consideration to minority students seeking admission to American medical colleges, similar programs should be developed to allow rural residents to be trained as physicians.

Certain manifestations of managed care, such as Medicare health maintenance organizations (HMOs), may soon become commonplace in urban locations. Insofar as such programs would be disastrous to the financial well-being of many rural medical practices that cater to a high percentage of elderly patients, rural physicians and residents can be further helped by not being forced out of traditional fee-for-service programs.

The rural areas of our nation are blessed with many physicians who are happy to live in the country and practice the unique type of medicine such locations require. Newspaper articles about young, idealistic physicians who set up medical practices in out-of-the-way places don't even begin to tell the real story of rural medicine or give politicians sufficient reason to ensure a greater measure of financial security for those who practice the art.

Rural physicians don't need strawberry sundaes to survive. Some scrambled eggs will do just fine - and maybe a few extra strips of bacon!

February, 1995

HOLDING YOUR BREATH

On June 20, 1997, the attorney general of Mississippi announced 40 states had reached an historic agreement with the tobacco industry. In a nationally-televised press conference, the visibly emotional attorney general briefly outlined a plan that would allow the tobacco industry help the states pay for the medical costs of tobacco-related illnesses in exchange for removal of 40 class action suits brought about by the states against the tobacco industry, as well as limited immunity from future lawsuits.

To be sure, the agreement caught many analysts off guard. Instead of the originally proposed $200 billion settlement by the tobacco industry and its agreement to send Joe Camel packing, the tobacco industry agreed to cough up $368 billion over the next 25 years, and consent to a myriad of potentially self-destructive provisions.

In addition to the punitive damages that would theoretically be used by the states to fund Medicaid, health programs for needy children, anti-smoking campaigns and addiction research, compensate injured smokers and sporting events that lose tobacco sponsors, and develop programs to help smokers kick the habit, the tobacco industry also agreed to dramatically curtail its own advertising and even pay for various anti-tobacco campaigns and programs. Additionally, the tobacco industry agreed to stock tobacco products behind store counters, eliminate cigarette vending machines, eliminate tobacco ads from billboards and signs, advertise cigarettes in black and white text rather than through the use of human images like the Marlboro Man or cartoon characters like Joe Camel, and eliminate advertising on the internet, product placement in movies, and the display of brand names and logos on such merchandise as athletic equipment, beach paraphernalia, and clothing.

What's more, the tobacco industry also agreed to give regulatory authority over tobacco products to the Food and Drug Administration (FDA) that could eventually mandate the elimination of nicotine and other addictive or harmful ingredients from tobacco products. The tobacco industry also agreed to print warning labels, such as: "Smoking can become addictive," "Smoking can cause cancer," and "Smoking can kill you," on packs of cigarettes, disclose all ingredients and additives in tobacco products, and make available any present and future data on nicotine addiction and other medical consequences of tobacco use.

Finally, the tobacco industry agreed to cooperate with the prohibition of smoking in public places and development of programs that would discourage the use of tobacco products by American youth. To this end, the tobacco industry agreed to fund the enforcement of such programs by the FDA and state authorities, and pay dramatically increased penalties for violations of FDA rules.

In exchange for these concessions, 40 states agreed to drop their class action suits against the tobacco industry. If and when these suits are dropped, the individual plaintiffs will receive no cash awards but will be eligible for smoking cessation help.

Pending private lawsuits against the tobacco industry would not be affected by this agreement, nor would the pending class action suit brought about by airline flight attendants because of illnesses caused by exposure to second-hand smoke. Although this agreement would prohibit future class action suits against the tobacco industry, individuals could still file private lawsuits and collect compensatory damages for expenses, lost wages, and pain and suffering, but not punitive damages for past industry misconduct.

President Clinton has promised to slowly and carefully peruse the 70-page agreement between the 40 states and the tobacco industry before offering any comments, and

Senate Majority Leader Trent Lott of Mississippi has announced Congress will start to formally study the agreement in September. Such political stalling techniques, of course, mean the President and the Congress plan to observe America's reactions to the tobacco accord before going on record with their own proclamations.

Insofar as 1,000 Americans continue to die each day from tobacco-related illnesses, and Americans have had the past 32 years to read the Surgeon General's warning on cigarette packs, it would appear America is finally starting to understand the dire consequences of tobacco use, as well as the wisdom of drastically curtailing, if not totally eliminating, such use. This contention is further supported by the fact that 1 out of every 2 Americans used tobacco products at the end of World War II while only 1 out of 4 Americans currently indulge in tobacco use.

It would seem logical, therefore, that most Americans would be in favor of the tobacco accord and would urge the President and Congress to approve the deal post haste. Given the peculiarities and nuances of politics, however, what are the odds that logic, common sense, and idealism will ultimately triumph?

Will the President and Congress be listening to the millions of Americans who have been imploring the removal of tobacco smoke from public air for the past 3 decades? Or will the folks in Washington be listening to louder and more influential voices who have grown accustomed to the aroma of tobacco in the air and who continue to profit from the use of tobacco by Americans?

Whose voice will be louder? Will it be the unified voice of a health-conscious America or the combined voices of the 45 million Americans who are still addicted to cigarettes; the farmers who make 10-times more money growing tobacco than vegetables; those who earn their living by converting tobacco into cigarettes, cigars, and chew; those who advertise tobacco products; those in the publishing, sports, and entertainment industries who rely on the support and sponsorship of the tobacco industry; the owners of the retail stores in which tobacco products account for over 25% of all sales; the owners of billboard and sign companies that owe their existence to tobacco; the owners of vending machine companies that dispense tobacco products; the civil liberties lawyers who continue to defend the right of Americans to smoke in public; the trial lawyers who are about to become involved in decades of tobacco-related lawsuits; and the investors who stand to profit from continued tobacco sales?

Whose voice will the politicians ultimately listen to? Will it be the gentle voice of concern or the discordant voice of special interest?

On June 20, 1997, forty states reached an agreement with the tobacco industry. It will be a long time before any of the provisions of the agreement are ever enacted into law, however, so, don't hold your breath!

On second thought, hold your breath, if you like. It's probably no more dangerous than breathing the smoke-filled air.

August, 1997

CLEARING THE AIR

When the attorney general of Mississippi recently announced 40 states had reached an historic agreement with the tobacco industry, he left many observers with the impression the agreement was a done deal. Nothing could be farther from the truth.

What the attorney general and his colleagues handed the American people on June 20, 1997 was a 2-ton slab of marble from which a 16-ounce figurine is about to be carved. Insofar as sculptures take time to complete and the process is complicated when more than one sculptor decides to work on the piece at the same time, don't expect any real tobacco deal any time soon.

If you're confused by the terms of the agreement that was recently promulgated between the states and the tobacco industry, just keep in mind the deal's bottom line. In essence, the tobacco industry has agreed to pay twice its current domestic profits each year for the next 25 years and sponsor programs and campaigns that promise to destroy the American tobacco culture in exchange for the removal of current class action suits against the tobacco industry and immunity from future class action suits.

Although the armchair quarterbacks have officially deemed the transaction an attempt by the tobacco industry to put a cap on its current and future liability, a few pertinent questions remain unanswered. First of all, how can an industry that expects to make $8.4 billion in domestic profits in 1998 agree to pay $15 billion dollars each year for the next quarter-century and, at the same time, sponsor programs designed to drastically curtail the use of tobacco products by Americans?

What's more, will the projected 75-cent increase in the cost of a pack of cigarettes, the continued irrational exuberance of those who invest in tobacco stocks, and even a ton of product liability insurance be able to save an industry that has essentially agreed to self-destruct? The answer to these questions, of course, is a resounding, "NO!"

The American tobacco industry hasn't gotten where it is today by not understanding how to take care of business. Pure and simple, the tobacco industry entered into its recent agreement with the states for no other purpose than to buy time.

By tentatively agreeing to pay unrealistic sums of money to the states and engage in all kinds of self-destructive programs, the tobacco industry realized it could take a breather from all its court activity and bad publicity, give smokers and those who profit from the sale of tobacco products a chance to make some noise, and closely observe how the courts handled a number of other pending class action suits involving product liability. If, for example, the Supreme Court failed to uphold Amchem Products versus Windsor, a class action suit that would limit the rights of future claimants who develop asbestos-related illnesses, the probability of the tobacco industry's being able to successfully defend itself in similar class action suits would dramatically increase.

The tobacco industry appeared to succumb to the wishes of the states and run away from its recent fight for no other purpose than to buy time to regroup and effectively live to fight another day. Before the tobacco industry's tentative agreement with the states can be adopted, it must first be approved by the President and Congress.

For starters, there is little question that, in his quest to be politically correct, Bill Clinton will approve some sort of tobacco agreement, but it won't be the same agreement he was handed. The President's many advisors will undoubtedly remind him of America' s longstanding tobacco heritage, tobacco's current role in our economy, and the ominous reality of Prohibition, black markets, and international trade deficits.

His advisors will also remind the President of the right of Americans to smoke as well as their option not to smoke, the inherent dangers of allowing a federal agency, such as the Food and Drug Administration, to be given too much control over factors that influence the lives of millions of Americans, and the perceived abandonment of the tobacco-growing states and their industry by William Jefferson Clinton and the Democratic Party.

Accordingly, the President will approve some sort of tobacco agreement, but it won't be any accord that authorizes the tobacco industry to self-destruct. From a large slab of marble, the President will help create a mere figurine.

Similarly, in its own quest to be understood and loved by all, Congress will also smoke the current tobacco agreement until there is nothing left but a few butts and some ashes. When the smoke has finally cleared and the final congressman has reminded us that expecting the tobacco industry to cough up $368 billion is cruel and unusual punishment and, as such, a direct violation of the tobacco industry's constitutional rights under the Eighth Amendment, very few people will remember the original terms of the tobacco accord.

Congressmen represent their constituents, and 45 million smokers and scads of other Americans who earn their living from tobacco don't want America to kick its smoking habit any time soon. Congress, too, will help create a figurine.

When the President and Congress finally get through with the tobacco agreement and each state finally get around to reviewing, debating, and signing the agreement, the courts will finally get their chance to host a seemingly endless array of legal challenges to the accord. Conceivably, every provision of any tobacco agreement could be challenged in court, especially provisions that limit the awards to plaintiffs with tobacco-related illnesses and provisions that restrict future lawsuits against the tobacco industry.

Court battles take time, as do appeals to higher courts and the final consideration of any matter by the Supreme Court. Such legal extravaganzas also require a great deal of financing.

Ergo, don't expect any final tobacco agreement any time soon. What's more, don't expect any final tobacco accord to be reached without the financial help of the great American taxpayer.

The tobacco industry realizes all the complexities involved in reaching meaningful and enforceable agreements between government and industry. The tobacco industry also realizes full many a contingency plan can be formulated while presidents, congresses, and courts argue over the wording of documents.

So, if and when a tobacco deal is ever finalized, the tobacco industry will already be 2 steps ahead of those who think they have forced the industry into compliance. Be it through increased international tobacco marketing, corporate restructuring, or bankruptcy and reorganization, the tobacco industry will be ready and able to carry on business as usual.

In the meantime, 1,000 Americans will die from tobacco-related illnesses and 3,000 new kids will be given the opportunity to start their own smoking habits each day. How many more lives will be lost or imperiled before America finally realizes it is no longer June 20, 1997, and the air we breathe is still not clear of tobacco's deadly stench?

August, 1997

ANTHRAX

On December 19, 1998, just hours after the United States had completed its most recent bombing of Iraq, officials were warned anthrax spores had been released into the air ducts of a federal building in Los Angeles. Ninety-one people who worked in the building were detained and observed for eight hours until FBI investigators and health officials were able to conclude deadly anthrax particles had not been dispersed through the building's ventilation system.

Anthrax, of course, is not a disease that normally lurks in air ducts and affects human beings. Instead, it is an infectious disease that normally affects livestock on farms and ranches.

Although the spread of anthrax has been effectively controlled by animal vaccination programs, the disease continues to affect livestock in areas of the world where such inoculation programs have not been successfully implemented. If terrorists have their way, however, anthrax could start to occur in areas of the world that have been targeted for biological warfare, and start to destroy human, rather than animal, populations.

When it comes to biological warfare, anthrax is the weapon of choice. Materials created from the naturally occurring bacterium, *Bacillus anthracis*, are extremely lethal, easy to produce in large quantities, relatively inexpensive to make, easy to incorporate into weapons, and difficult to detect. Anthrax is extremely stable and can be stored indefinitely as a dry powder, freeze-dried or aerosolized.

When it is inhaled by unprotected and unvaccinated people, anthrax is frequently fatal. On a per gram basis, anthrax is 100,000 times deadlier than the deadliest chemical warfare agent.

A single gram of anthrax can yield 100-million lethal doses. Humans can acquire anthrax by handling infected animal hides and contracting the bacteria through cuts in the skin, by eating infected meat or by inhaling anthrax spores.

Although localized cutaneous anthrax can occasionally regress to a systemic infection and lead to death, and gastrointestinal anthrax can cause a debilitating enteritis and result in death in a high percentage of cases, these forms of the disease can usually be treated effectively with antibiotics such as: penicillin, erythromycin, tetracycline, chloramphenicol and ciprofloxacin.

Inhalational anthrax, on the other hand, is frequently fatal in unprotected and unvaccinated people. Symptoms of inhalational anthrax usually begin one to six days following exposure, are usually non-specific and typically include a low-grade fever, dry hacking cough and weakness.

Those infected with inhalational anthrax may appear to improve following a two to four-day flu-like illness, only to develop respiratory distress, go into shock and die within the next 24 hours, regardless of treatment. It is this initial flu-like appearance of anthrax, as well as its atypical clinical course, that make the disease difficult to diagnose and equally difficult to treat.

For these and many other valid reasons, anthrax has become the preferred agent of biological warfare. In addition to Iraq, which has previously declared possession of 9,000 liters of anthrax, nine other foreign countries are thought to be developing anthrax weapons in their biological warfare programs.

What's more, other groups are thought to be developing anthrax weapons within the borders of the United States. In recent months, abortion clinics in four midwestern states have received anthrax threats.

Understandably, our Defense Department and law enforcement agencies have been concerned about anthrax for quite some time. Nowhere is this concern more apparent than in the Department of Defense's recent anthrax vaccine initiative.

During the 1991 Persian Gulf War, for example, more than 150,000 American troops and 3,000 special operations personnel received anthrax vaccinations. A $130 million military inoculation program is currently underway and expected to finish vaccinating all active duty and reserve military personnel by the year 2005.

The anthrax vaccine that is currently being used by the Defense Department has been licensed by the Food and Drug Administration (FDA) since 1970, and is a cell-free filtrate vaccine, or one that uses dead rather than live bacteria. Although the anthrax vaccine is currently being manufactured for use mainly by military personnel, it has been made available to veterinarians, lab workers and livestock handlers for the past quarter-century and, during that time, has been recommended for use by healthy, non-pregnant 18- to 65-year-olds.

It is apparent biological warfare has become a reality and a foreign enemy could very easily bring anthrax into the United States, mass produce anthrax-laden materials within our borders, and disseminate deadly anthrax particles through American air. In the earliest stages, mass anthrax inhalation in a major metropolitan area could be misinterpreted as a flu epidemic and, by the time anthrax was finally diagnosed, the lives of millions of Americans could be lost.

This being the case, it would seem prudent for the federal government to provide citizens with anthrax vaccine. Unfortunately, immunizing America against anthrax is not as easy as it might seem.

For starters, the current anthrax vaccine is given as three subcutaneous injections two weeks apart, followed by three additional injections at six, twelve and eighteen months. Yearly boosters are required to maintain immunity.

Although temporary side effects from the anthrax vaccine are usually mild and similar to those from flu shots, six separate inoculations over a period of eighteen months are required to assure immunity. However, some protection against the disease is believed to be provided following the first 3 vaccinations.

Partial protection against anthrax following the first three vaccinations is supported by the finding anthrax vaccine given to Rhesus monkeys at zero and two weeks is 100% effective in preventing disease following aerosol challenges at eight and thirty-eight-weeks. Obviously, there are many separate health factors that determine the immunologic response of each individual given anthrax vaccine.

Even if a mass inoculation program were to be started at this very moment in the United States, Americans would still be months away from developing complete immunity to anthrax. Obviously, a lot can happen in several months, but there are significant numbers of military personnel, federal officials and scientists who seem to think American citizens, including those in
the military, would be better off without the anthrax vaccine.

The internet is laden with condemnations of the anthrax vaccine from military personnel who attribute their Gulf War Syndrome to either anthrax vaccine used alone or in combination with other vaccines. In response, vaccine use has been publicly defended by the Surgeon General of the U.S. Army, as well as the Presidential Advisory Committee on Gulf War Veteran's Illnesses.

In 1996, this committee concluded it was unlikely anthrax vaccine used alone or in combination with botulinum toxoid caused the health effects sustained by Gulf War veterans who were engaged in Operation Desert Storm. In its report, the committee cited various researches that have documented the safety of administering multiple simultaneous immunizations.

It is significant to note the allegations of anthrax vaccine causing the symptoms of Gulf War Syndrome are not supported by the experience with the vaccine in the private sector. For over a quarter-century, thousands of veterinarians, lab workers and livestock handlers have been given the anthrax vaccine without any reports of the chronic fatigue, arthralgias, rashes, dyspnea, hair loss, diarrhea, insomnia, attention and memory deficits, nightmares or night sweats that are seen in patients with Gulf War Syndrome.

The internet has also posted various articles that challenge the safety and efficacy of anthrax vaccine and question the practices of the vaccine's manufacturer. A number of these articles describe various warning letters that the manufacturer received from the FDA concerning quality control issues.

Although it is true the anthrax vaccine's manufacturer has received a number of letters relative to quality control concerns by the FDA, the vaccine appears to have enjoyed a good safety record in the private sector since 1970. In limited numbers of human efficacy studies and greater numbers of animal studies, the vaccine appeared to be effective in preventing both cutaneous and inhalational anthrax.

Finally, the internet has published the condemnations of vaccines in general and the anthrax vaccine in particular by various physicians and scientists. The presence of impurities in the anthrax vaccine has been widely discussed as has been the propensity for certain vaccines to lead to serious autoimmune diseases.

Although impurities do occur in vaccines and these impurities can lead to side-effects, both impurities and side-effects have been decreased by improved vaccine production techniques. Although there appears to be a cause-and-effect relationship between certain vaccines and a number of serious autoimmune disorders, the incidence of such disorders in vaccinated individuals is believed to be very low.

It is obvious the population of the United States could be decimated by anthrax at any time. It is also obvious the United States is not currently prepared to handle such a potential catastrophe.

We may be able to slow down the biological warfare program of any foreign country with surgical air strikes, but bombs alone are incapable of totally eliminating such programs. High tech labs, large sums of money and classified research papers are not among the things that are required to mass produce anthrax.

The day may come when the entire world finally learns to live in peace. Unfortunately, today is not that day.

Until the world discovers peace, the United States must continue to defend itself against foreign aggression. As it pertains to 1999, the United States must find a way to protect itself against anthrax.

A consensus of available research findings would seem to support the safety and efficacy of the current anthrax vaccine. To become practical, however, the vaccine would have to be redesigned to provide complete immunity against anthrax with fewer injections, in a much shorter period of time and with an added margin of safety.

If it has not already done so, the federal government needs to sponsor research that would lead to the development of a practical anthrax vaccine and the means for making such a vaccine available to the American people. At the same time, the federal government also needs to sponsor research that would lead to the development of effective post-exposure treatment for inhalational anthrax – especially anthrax anti-toxin, as well as rapid screening tests that could detect anthrax in a single drop of blood or expectorated sputum within a few minutes time.

Not that many years ago, Americans built bomb shelters to protect themselves against nuclear warfare. The time has come for Americans to understand our current enemies are not as likely to drop nuclear bombs from the sky as they are to disperse agents of biological warfare into the air we breathe.

If for no other reason than to deter the continued development of biological warfare by our enemies, anthrax vaccine should be made available to every American. The threat of biological warfare is real. If the threat wasn't real, non-combat military personnel and National Guardsmen wouldn't be currently lining up to receive their anthrax shots.

March, 1999

THE CLEAR AND PRESENT
DANGER OF ANTHRAX

Bioterrorism is a clear and present danger to the United States. Anthrax remains the weapon of choice of bioterrorists, and it will as long as Americans continue to believe the misinformation self-proclaimed experts are currently disseminating on television.

For the record, it is improbable bioterrorists will fly a blimp filled with anthrax into the Super Bowl. What is more probable is that terrorists will try to infect small to moderate numbers of people at multiple sites in different geographic locales by transmitting anthrax spores through ventilation systems or biological letter bombs.

In 1966, the U.S. Army released *Bacillus globigii*, an anthrax simulant, into New York City subway tubes and allowed convection caused by trains to aerosolize the endospores. Follow-up studies clearly demonstrated thousands of people could have been exposed to lethal doses of anthrax in the same fashion, and creating an effective biological weapon is not as difficult as previously thought.

In 1979, less than one gram of anthrax was accidentally released from a biological weapons facility in Sverdlovsk, USSR. Of the thousands who were exposed to anthrax, 66 died but 11 survived following aggressive treatment with anti-anthrax globulin, antibiotics including penicillin, cephalosporins and chloramphenicol, and steroids.

None of the vaccinated facility workers acquired anthrax and a massive public health response, utilizing immunization, prophylactic tetracycline, and the disinfection of homes and paving of unpaved streets, stopped spread of the disease. However, seven sheep and one cow being raised in an anthrax-free environment 50 kilometers downwind of the facility died from anthrax within a few days of the accident.

This episode clearly disproves that large quantities of anthrax are required to infect large populations, many spores must be inhaled before anthrax can occur, immediate medical treatment following anthrax exposure is 100% effective in preventing fatalities, ciprofloxacin is the only antibiotic effective in the treatment or prophylaxis of anthrax, and every strain of anthrax is quickly and completely destroyed by the environment. Although the LD-50, or lethal dose of anthrax required to kill 50% of the population, is 8,000-10,000 spores, mathematical models have shown as little as nine spores could have infected susceptible Sverdlovsk residents.

Recently, a Florida resident died of inhalational anthrax. Initial reports implicated anthrax acquired from a North Carolina stream.

In multiple studies, Rhesus monkeys could not be infected with anthrax through drinking water. Taking this into account, as well as the sophistication of America's water treatment plants, bioterrorism using water as a delivery system seems highly unlikely.

Finally, government officials and CDC spokesmen recently stated anthrax vaccine is not being given to U.S. citizens or military personnel because six inoculations over 18 months are required for immunity. Two separate observations make this information suspect.

First, anthrax vaccine given to Rhesus monkeys at zero and two weeks is 100% effective in preventing disease following aerosol challenges at eight and thirty-eight weeks. Second, the Department of Defense previously ordered use of the current anthrax vaccine to immunize all active duty and reserve military personnel by the year 2005.

Extended dosing is not a reason to withhold anthrax vaccine. Unavailability, lack of safety or ineffectiveness of the vaccine could be.

At this very moment, the danger of anthrax in America is clear and present. Our response requires a safe vaccine, effective anti-toxin, and injection of real experts into television news programming.

November, 2001

DESELECTION

A young sailor at sea aboard an aircraft carrier was phoned by his wife and informed she had given birth to twins. The sailor was also informed his older dimwitted brother had renewed a longstanding family tradition and named the newborns in his absence.

"What did my brother name our little girl?" the sailor asked.

"Denise," his wife replied.

"Why, that's alright," the sailor acknowledged with a sigh of relief. "And what did he name our little boy?"

After a short pause, the wife replied, "Denephew!"

Just as the sailor was surprised to learn of a new son with an unusual name, an inordinately large number of American physicians have been surprised to learn of their deselection from managed care. Deselection, of course, is the termination of a physician's contract by a managed care program.

Insofar as many physicians have not openly confessed their deselection because of fears of similar actions by other insurers, potential litigation or lost confidence by patients and colleagues, the exact number of physicians who have been deselected is currently unknown. It has been conservatively estimated, however, that tens of thousands of American physicians have been deselected by managed care programs since 1992.

As managed care programs have entered new markets, they have vigorously recruited any and all physicians who have been willing to join the program and accept the program's many provisions - including the program's right to terminate a physician without cause. After many managed care programs have assembled impressive lists of participating physicians and used these lists to lure patients into the poorly understood realm of managed care, they have quickly deselected those physicians perceived as liabilities.

Physicians with below-average professional skills or work habits; histories of malpractice or professional sanctions; propensities for ordering above-average numbers of tests, consultations or treatments; sub-optimal popularity with patients, colleagues or professional staff; or attitudes or philosophies incompatible with those of managed care have been generally perceived as liabilities by managed care programs. Accordingly, such physicians have been among the first to undergo the process of deselection.

In general, managed care programs have not been especially grateful for the hundreds of patients any physician has brought into a managed care network or particularly moved by the desire of such a physician to remain in the network. Accordingly, managed care programs have not shown a great deal of compassion when it comes to physician deselection.

Similarly, managed care programs have not shown a great deal of understanding when it comes to the special needs of their patients. Physicians who have treated large numbers of crippled and disabled patients, for example, have been deselected because they have ordered above-average numbers of tests and treatments for patients whose health could not be adequately maintained by any physician without above-average numbers of tests and treatments.

Simply put, managed care wants its physicians to be happy campers who are willing and able to do more for less. Physicians who do not fit such a profile are deselections waiting for a place to happen.

To date, the vast majority of physician deselections have been terminations without cause - a provision accepted, sometimes unwittingly, by physicians contracting with managed care programs. This provision has given managed care programs the license to terminate the contract of any physician for any reason without so much as the courtesy of an explanation.

Prior to 1997, only eight states required managed care programs to provide a written explanation to deselected physicians, and only six states required managed care programs to provide deselected physicians with a formal appeals process. Current activity in the courts and legislatures, however, should stop this trend and lead to the legislation of greater managed care accountability in the not-too-distant future.

Due to a tremendous number of lawsuits brought against managed care programs by deselected physicians, managed care has recently done an about-face and started providing explanations to deselected physicians, or terminating such physicians "with cause." To be sure, managed care programs have not decided to apprise physicians of the reason for their termination because it is the ethical or decent thing to do; instead, managed care programs have adopted this policy because of recent court experience demonstrating it is much less expensive to defend a case of termination with cause in court than it is to defend a case involving termination without cause.

To understand physician deselection is to understand the folly that is managed care. The raison d'etre of managed care is to control as much of our one-trillion-dollar health care industry as possible and, in doing so, to lavish untold wealth on managed care's purveyors, supporters and facilitators.

Managed care is not concerned with how little health care patients can be made to accept or how many professional reputations are destroyed in the process. Managed care is only concerned with generating megabucks at the expense of patients and physicians.

In addition to demonstrating the strength of managed care, the process of deselection has also clearly demonstrated the weakness of organized medicine in America. Managed care has effectively thrown tens of thousands of physicians out into the cold with little more than token resistance from the so-called leadership of the American medical profession.

Additionally, managed care has attempted to replace the most sophisticated and resourceful health care delivery system in the history of mankind with a system where health care is rationed to millions of Americans. This, too, has met little more than token resistance from medicine's power elite.

Fortunately, what goes around, comes around, and America is finally starting to wake up to the reality of managed care. With each new passing day, more Americans are leaving managed care and returning to conventional health care, more employers are canceling managed care contracts, and more legislators are coming to the realization managed care is a folly that has never been and could never be in America's best interest.

More physicians are also starting to realize they don't need to belong to a managed care network to run their medical practice or earn a comfortable living. They are also starting to realize a surprising number of patients will change their health insurance for no other reason than to be able to see the physician of their choice.

Managed care's days are numbered, and the time has come for physicians to do unto managed care what managed care would surely do unto them. The process is called deselection - and it works both ways!

September, 1997

VICARIOUS DESELECTION

Deselection is the process whereby a physician's contract with a managed care program is terminated - usually without explanation or rights of appeal. Since 1992, tens of thousands of American physicians have been deselected by managed care programs.

To be formally deselected, a physician must first participate in a managed care program. Through the process of "vicarious deselection," however, even physicians who refuse to participate in managed care can be publicly embarrassed by the very programs they have chosen to avoid.

Recently, a working man was informed his company was changing health insurance and switching to managed care. When he reviewed the new health plan's roster of participating physicians, he realized his primary care physician was not on the list.

Insofar as his company had opted for a "point of service" health insurance program, the employee was told he and his family could continue to receive medical services from their primary care physician and his company's new health plan would reimburse 70% of the cost of such services. Reluctant to receive only 70% reimbursement when his fellow employees were receiving full reimbursement for the services received from the company's health maintenance organization, he wrote the following letter to the administrator of his company's new health plan:

"This letter is to request that my family's physician of 12 years be appointed our personal primary care physician. He is not on your health plan's list of participating physicians but, due to extenuating circumstances, it is imperative that we do not change physicians.

"We live in a rural area 50 miles from the county where most of your participating physicians practice medicine. A few of these physicians have offices in our county, but they are unable to provide the comprehensive medical services that we currently receive from our own doctor. Also, our doctor can be easily reached 7 days a week and he makes house calls when necessary.

"I have 3 herniated discs in my back due to a work-related injury. On 4 occasions, I had to contact our doctor at odd hours for immediate treatment. The last time, 3 years ago, I was taken to the doctor's office by ambulance. Within 11/2 hours of the time of injury, I was in the hospital getting medical care without a hassle from some ER doctor who didn't understand my complicated medical history.

"Our daughter has had chronic otitis media since she was 3 years old. Her hearing was 25% at that time. An ear specialist at a large medical center wanted to put tubes in her ears without even examining her. When we consulted our doctor, he advised medical treatment rather than tubes. Today, at the age of 12, our daughter has 96% hearing, is an honor student, and is in the school band. Our doctor helped us avoid an unnecessary operation.

"My wife has many complicated medical problems. She is in a wheelchair because of an amputation, has crippling arthritis and multiple herniated discs, as well as vascular problems, peptic ulcer disease, and frequent infections. It is very difficult for her to get around and she experiences constant pain. Also, being a brittle diabetic, she needs a physician she can contact at a moment's notice. Many a time our doctor has had to be called in the middle of the night to attend to her. Because he knows her complete medical history, he can usually advise my wife over the phone on what to do, making a trip to the hospital unnecessary. Also, when injections for pain and inflammation are warranted, our doctor can do them right in his office without having to send my wife to a specialist or to the hospital.

"If we have to switch to a primary care physician on your list, many specialists will have to be contacted and used on a frequent basis. This will be a major problem for us and expensive for you.

"Please give this appeal your grave consideration. It is a very major problem. We need our doctor."

Two weeks later, the worker received the following reply from the administrator of his company's new health plan:

"In response to your recent letter, I have reviewed the information and certainly understand your concern.

"As you know, we are a managed care organization composed of a network of participating primary care and specialist physicians.
In order to be a participating physician in the network, physicians must be certified by the Quality Management Committee. This assures that our members receive quality care. Exceptions cannot be made to this policy as this could put our quality of care at risk.

"Insofar as we only deal with providers who we certify (who pass our quality standards and are participating), we will not provide coverage for continuation of care for your family by your current physician. Please contact us if we can assist you in selecting a participating primary care physician."

In addition to deselecting physicians who have contracted with their programs, managed care also employs vicarious deselection to insidiously damage the reputations of physicians who have refused to join managed care networks. The reply you've just read illustrates how vicarious deselection works.

With such a carefully-phrased reply, managed care programs indirectly question the abilities and credentials of physicians who do not participate in their network. Such replies conveniently disregard the ease with which any

91

physician can be certified to participate in a managed care plan, and attempt to obfuscate a physician's distaste for managed care with some ill-defined professional impairment.

Once a managed care program has confused a patient about the "quality" of his or her physician, it is easy to use its two-tier reimbursement system to destroy a solid, oftentimes long-standing, doctor-patient relationship. This, of course, frequently forces the patient into managed care by default.

Managed care programs usually accomplish this task by reimbursing 100% of the medical services obtained within a managed care network but only 70% of the services obtained outside the network. As might be expected, payment for services obtained outside the managed care network is generally made slowly and not without an inordinate number of claim rejections, requests for additional information and multiple repeat billings.

With time, many patients grow tired of paying for 30% of their medical care and continually fighting for the 70% payment promised but not delivered by their managed care plan. If the physician starts complaining about slow reimbursement, predictable friction between the patient and physician usually ensues, frequently forcing patients into the land of managed care where medical services are "free" and obtained without hassle!

The same politically-protected health care system that has been allowed to deselect physicians without explanation or recourse has also been sanctioned to vicariously deselect physicians who have refused to participate in managed care. Gag orders, anyone?

September, 1997

DRUNK DRIVING

My youngest son and I were midway through our late-night dinner when the phone rang.

"Dad, I don't want you to worry," my daughter said with characteristic poise, "but Mom and I were just in a serious accident. A drunk driver swerved into our car from the opposite lane and hit us broadside. It's a good thing we were wearing our seat belts."

"Honey, are you and Mom alright?" I asked with great concern.

"Yeah, Dad, we're okay," my daughter answered. "Mom has bruises over her ribs and we're both a little shaken, but we're alright. I wish I could say the same for our car, though. The car is toast."

"Don't worry about the car," I said, in a tone of voice meant to convey understanding. "Was the other driver hurt?"

"I don't think so," my daughter replied, "but I'm not sure because he drove off. Dad, he never even stopped to see if we were hurt."

Instructing my daughter to call the police, I immediately left home and made my way to the accident site. As I drove along the dark country roads, I thought about what my wife and daughter were going through.

Having been hit broadside by a drunk driver myself, I understood the state of shock my loved ones were experiencing. Having treated hundreds of patients who were the innocent victims of drunk driving, I understood the mixed emotions my wife and daughter were feeling.

When I arrived at the accident site, I immediately comforted my wife and daughter, and listened to the gruesome details of the criminal act that had transpired. When I inspected the demolished remains of what was once a handsome Chrysler Imperial, I realized the survival of my wife and daughter truly bordered on the miraculous.

After a young state trooper completed his inspection of our wreck and dislodged pieces of the other car for evidence, I inquired about his plans for locating the inebriated hit-and-run artist. The trooper replied he planned to visit the parking lots of a few local bars to see if he could spot any damaged cars.

When I asked if he planned to send a description of the other driver's vehicle to local garages and body shops, he informed me such measures were only employed under certain circumstances. When I asked if someone had to be killed or maimed for the police to consider an accident a certain circumstance, the trooper offered no comment.

We continue to have a serious problem with drunk driving in the United States today because we are content to wait until someone is killed or seriously injured before we decide to bring drunk drivers to justice. We wait for the crash, the screams and the sirens before we decide to whip out the breathalyzer and tell the drunk driver what he already knows.

Drunks need to be kept out of their cars and off our roads before they destroy life and limb. Cleaning up after the inevitable accident happens and punishing the drunk offender post facto is as short-sighted as closing the proverbial barn door after the horse has already left.

The states decide which restaurants and bars will be licensed to sell alcoholic beverages, and it is the prerogative of the states to establish rules and regulations that control the sale of liquor. The states could take a giant step toward eliminating drunk driving by exercising greater control over the sale of alcoholic beverages.

For example, the liquor control boards of each state could mandate the use of breathalyzers in restaurants and bars licensed to sell alcoholic beverages. Patrons who appeared to be inebriated could be asked to have the alcohol content of their breath voluntarily analyzed before they left the establishment in the interest of public safety.

Those who agreed to take the breathalyzer test and whose results were abnormal could have alternate transportation arranged by the management of the restaurant or bar. In cases involving inebriated patrons who refused to be tested with a breathalyzer or who insisted on driving away drunk, police could be notified by the restaurant or bar management with immunity from legal reprisals guaranteed by law.

The use of breathalyzers in restaurants and bars, of course, is not about to happen any time soon. The reason has very little to do with impracticality or inconvenience but a whole lot to do with our national reverence for the almighty dollar.

Restaurants and bars make much more money selling booze than food. In fact, various national restaurant chains have been accused of intentionally building undersized facilities for no other reason than to promote the sale of more booze.

When popular restaurants are small and reservations are not taken, diners frequently have to wait inordinate amounts of time for their tables. When diners are forced to wait for their tables, they can usually be coaxed to do their waiting over a few drinks.

The sale of alcoholic beverages accounts for megabucks in America and any business or industry that generates megabucks can usually garner the support of a slew of politicians. Consequently, the protection of business or industry is a greater priority to certain legislators than is the promotion of public safety.

At this very moment, drunks are driving out of restaurant and bar parking lots all over the United States. At this very moment, innocent Americans are losing life and limb in motor vehicle accidents caused by drunk drivers.

There are ways to stop such senseless crime. Unfortunately, the powers-that-be are unwilling to employ the necessary measures.

At this very moment, someone is probably reading this essay and deciding that preventive measures designed to keep drunks off the road and obviate accidental death and injury would serve as an unwarranted threat to personal freedom by government. To such a reader, I would submit that the role of government is to govern, and the kind of person who would drive under the influence of alcohol, destroy valuable property, injure innocent people, leave the scene of a crime and repeat the same cycle at the earliest opportunity is in desperate need of being governed.

March, 1998

ELECTILE DYSFUNCTION

I had another one of those crazy dreams again last night. It was the third year of the presidential election recount in Florida and I was in Orlando covering the story for Newsweek.

Having tried unsuccessfully to determine the winner of Florida's 25 electoral votes and the presidency of the United States through legal, legislative and political channels, candidates George Bush and Al Gore finally agreed to personally poll each Florida resident. To accomplish this task, they agreed to ride together in a horse-drawn carriage through the streets of Florida at night and tally the votes residents cast by displaying lanterns in their homes.

The Florida residents seemed to like the idea of seeing their candidates up close and personal, and being able to display their electoral preferences in a manner consistent with historical tradition. As they eagerly awaited the appearance of the election carriage in their neighborhoods, Floridians prepared to vote one lantern if by Gore and two if by Bush to finally settle the Florida stalemate.

Accompanying Bush and Gore in the election carriage was Pat Buchanan who agreed to explain why any questionable or uncertain lantern votes belonged to Al Gore. Driving the carriage was Rain Man who had the reputation of being an excellent driver, a student of the People's Court and the one man who could be relied on to locate every street in Florida while keeping the election tally straight.

Following the election carriage through Florida was a caravan of double-decker buses. The buses were filled with politicians, lawyers, aides, reporters and a group of foreign tourists who hopped on the wrong bus and were still waiting to see the Empire State Building.

As the election carriage stopped for a red light, the candidates ran into a local McDonald's to use the restroom. The entire entourage also stormed the restaurant, prompting a counter girl to scream, "We got buses!"

As everyone within two city blocks ran toward McDonald's, Rain Man calmly got down from the carriage and approached his horse. "I'm an excellent driver," he whispered in the horse's ear.

"Hello, Rain Man," I said, as I approached the carriage.

"Hello," he replied. "Are you a doctor?"

"Why, yes, I am," I said. "How did you know?"

"You're wearing a white coat and you've got a stethoscope hanging around your neck," he answered.

"Yeah, but I only look like this when I'm dreaming," I replied.

"One potato, two potato, three potato, Gore," he mumbled.

"Rain Man, do you like the way this presidential election is going?" I inquired.

"No," he answered succinctly.

"How would the Rain Man run a presidential election?" I asked.

Without hesitation, Rain Man whispered into the horse's ear.

"Excuse me," the horse interjected. "My name is Mister Ed. I am the Rain Man's official spokesanimal and he's asked me to make the following brief statement on his behalf."

Clearing his throat, the talking horse continued. "After careful statistical analysis, Rain Man believes the presidential election process in the United States would be facilitated by mailing a uniform ballot to every American two weeks before the election deadline. The ballot should be similar to a standard test answer sheet with circles that can be filled in with a black pen and counted by optical recognition technology. The social security number of the voter, as well as a toll-free number that can be called for assistance with the voting procedure, should be imprinted on the ballot. The ballot should also be accompanied by a postage-paid envelope that is addressed to the independent accounting firm that will tabulate the votes."

Mister Ed cleared his voice again. "Once the ballot has been completed, it must be signed, dated and mailed before the election deadline. After the votes have been completely counted, each state will be notified of the results and each voter will be mailed a personal identification number, as well as a computerized printout of their votes. When included with their next income tax returns, these personal identification numbers will entitle voters to a $100 tax deduction. These numbers will also allow voters to confirm their identity in any communications with election boards. This process will ensure privacy, adequate time to study and submit a ballot, proof ballots were processed as per the intent of each voter, a system of checks and balances, greater reliability, the controlled announcement of election results and tax incentives to participate in the election process. The elimination of voting centers, equipment and personnel will result in savings to taxpayers."

Before I had the chance to ask any other questions, the candidates returned to the election carriage, their entourage returned to the buses, and Rain Man reclaimed his driver's seat.

"A doctor, named Samuel Prescott, rode with Paul Revere through Lexington and Concord on April 18, 1775," he said quietly, as he took the reins in his hands. "He was an excellent rider."

As Rain Man led the caravan away, Ralph Nader pulled up to the traffic light in a mint-condition Chevy Corvair.

"What are you doing here?" I asked.

"Collecting votes for the Green Party," he replied. "Gore gets all the houses with one lantern and Bush gets all those with two, but I get all the green traffic lights. Hey, there's another vote. Gotta go."

Just then, I awoke with a craving for a tall glass of orange juice and the realization electile dysfunction can be cured.

I've got to stop drinking shots of Jack Daniels and Lone Star chasers before I go to bed.

December, 2000

COMPETENCE

I recently perused a few of the diplomas, certificates and awards that adorn my office walls. The wording of these documents brought the issue of competence to mind.

My diploma from Temple University, for example, acknowledges that I received "the degree of Doctor of Medicine together with all the rights, privileges and honors appertaining thereto in recognition of the satisfactory completion of the course prescribed by the faculty of the university." My certificate from the American Board of Internal Medicine states that I have "met the requirements of this board," and have been "designated a Diplomate certified in the specialty of Internal Medicine."

My Pennsylvania medical license affirms that I, "having given satisfactory evidence of fitness as to age, character, preliminary education, medical instruction and all other matters required by law, was fully examined by the National Board of Medical Examiners and found duly qualified for the practice of medicine and surgery." Six separate American Medical Association (AMA) "Physician's Recognition Awards" attest to the fact that, for the past 18 years, I have continually "fulfilled the requirements for the Physician's Recognition Award in Continuing Medical Education."

Various and sundry other diplomas, educational certificates and professional awards also cover my office walls. All in all, they attest to a lifetime of education, training and dedication to the practice of medicine.

Once upon a time, diplomas, board certifications, medical licenses, continuing medical education certificates and professional honors were generally accepted as evidence of a physician's competence to practice medicine. Today, however, many of the same instigators who brought socialized medicine to America under the guise of managed care, are trying to convince Americans the competence of their physicians must be tested, retested and then tested all over again.

In an attempt to gain control over and personally profit from our $1 trillion health care industry, an interesting assortment of politicians, businessmen and legal eagles have schemed to create laws that favor the insurance industry and penalize the medical profession, discredit American physicians in the public eye and create the illusion America has such an overwhelming surplus of physicians that it can afford to pick and choose its caregivers. As a result, physicians have been eliminated from the medical profession in the malpractice courts, pressured out of medicine by health insurers and deselected from the very managed care organizations they helped create.

The purveyors of socialized medicine have successfully controlled the American medical profession in the courts, legislatures and news media. Defrocking a targeted group of physicians through bogus competency exams appears to be their next mission.

For the record, the American physician is more highly educated, more extensively trained and more thoroughly tested than any other professional in the entire world. Incompetent individuals occasionally fall through the cracks of medical education and become licensed to practice medicine, but the number of such individuals is not of sufficient magnitude to warrant the wholesale testing of the entire medical profession.

For the same record, incompetent physicians are individuals who lack the skill, knowledge or ability to practice medicine. They are not physicians who lose malpractice suits because of maloccurrence, physicians who are forced to render sub-optimal treatment because of the directives of managed care organizations, health insurers or other employers, or physicians who fail to win popularity contests.

Even if the competence of the American medical profession was a valid concern, the construction of a practical, unbiased and informative examination or set of examinations that could be administered to America's physicians would be a virtual impossibility. Not only would such examinations have to be specific for each medical and surgical specialty, but they would also have to be individualized to measure the unique characteristics of every physician's medical or surgical practice.

Insofar as the pathology and standards of practice differ greatly for internists who practice in the inner city, those who practice in a rural setting and those who practice somewhere in between, no one internal medicine exam could be used to measure the competence of internists who practice in different geographic locales and who treat different diseases. Internists might practice in a medical office, clinic, hospital, nursing facility, procedure unit, emergency department, academic center or any combination of locations and, because skill and knowledge requirements vary with location, no one examination could be used to measure the competence of internists working in such significantly different professional settings.

Even if an examination that truly measured physician competence could be constructed, the time and expense involved in preparing for and actually taking such a test would be a hardship for many physicians, as well as their families, patients and colleagues who provided patient coverage. Such hardship would be multiplied several-fold for those physicians who failed the exam and were labeled "incompetent" by the examination board.

Those who stand to profit from physician competency exams are already starting to count the megabucks to be earned from exam fees, preparation courses and numerous other related materials and services. Unfortunately, no one has begun to measure the downside potential of such exams.

What happens, for example, if a physician fails a competency exam? Does such a physician automatically forfeit his or her right to practice medicine until the test can be repeated?

What happens to the patients of physicians who have failed a competency exam? Are they supposed to find a new physician or just go without medical care until their physician can re-establish his or her competence through repeat testing?

What happens to the many patients who suddenly learn that their physician of thirty years has been deemed incompetent? Can such patients sue for malpractice because they received medical care from an incompetent physician?

What happens to a physician who fails a competency test but passes a retest? Can competence really be lost and then miraculously rediscovered a few weeks later at a new test site?

It is the responsibility of our medical schools and residency programs to teach physicians how to be competent. It is the responsibility of our specialty boards and state licensing boards to ensure that physician competence has been achieved through graduate and post-graduate training, and that it is maintained through approved programs of continuing medical education.

The medical profession already has more than enough checks and balances to ensure the competence of its members. One more examination will do little to ascertain or improve the competence of America's physicians.

Whenever I look at the many diplomas, certificates and awards that adorn my office walls, I realize how proud I am to be a member of a profession that has created the most sophisticated health care delivery system in the history of the world. I realize how fortunate I am to be in the company of so many competent colleagues.

April, 1999

HOSPITALISTS

In one of the early scenes from *Fiddler On The Roof*, a villager tells his neighbors he doesn't care about anything that happens outside their small community.

"Why should I break my head about the outside world?" he asks. "Let the outside world break its own head!"

In response, Tevye replies, "He's right!"

Hearing the villager, the young scholar, Perchik, argues to the contrary.

"You can't close your eyes to what's happening in the world," he observes.

Once again, Tevye replies, "He's right!"

When yet another villager comments that two men with contrasting opinions can't both be right, Tevye smiles and diplomatically concedes, "You know – you're also right!"

I am reminded of this scene from *Fiddler On The Roof* whenever I listen to the current debate about hospitalists. Hospitalists, of course, are physicians who manage the medical care of hospitalized patients.

In a sense, hospitalists are like medical residents who admit the patients of other physicians to the hospital, render the required medical treatment and then return the patients to their primary care physicians. Unlike medical residents, however, hospitalists are not physicians-in-training but duly licensed and certified physicians who are gainfully employed by hospitals or medical groups to practice in-patient medicine.

There are those who believe hospitalized patients should be managed by hospitalists. They argue hospitalized patients receive more efficient medical treatment from hospitalists, have shorter hospital stays and are more likely to have their health care managed in a cost-effective manner.

On the other hand, there are those who believe hospitalized patients should be managed by their personal physicians. This camp argues hospitalized patients feel more comfortable and secure with their own physicians, are less likely to receive incomplete treatment or be discharged prematurely and pose no real threat to the financial integrity of the health insurance industry.

The heated debate over who should manage hospitalized patients has met with the predictable response of those entrusted with the development of American health care policy. Much like Tevye, these politicians have agreed with fans of the hospitalist movement, agreed with defenders of a more traditional health care delivery system and even agreed with those who have accused them of trying to agree with everybody.

To be sure, the hospitalist concept is not one that should be quickly dismissed for lack of merit. The ability of a hospital to provide full-time, on-site physicians who are capable of rendering comprehensive in-patient care would help patients without personal physicians, patients whose personal physicians were unable to admit their patients to hospitals and patients whose medical emergencies did not permit the time to locate a personal physician or persuade an on-call physician to come to the hospital.

Just as the hospitalist concept would benefit many patients, it would also help many physicians. The ability to practice as a hospitalist would benefit physicians who preferred employment over the financial responsibilities of private practice, physicians whose professional interests were better satisfied in a hospital environment than in a medical office and physicians who required the security of a regular paycheck, guaranteed benefits and predictable scheduling.

The hospitalist concept would also help many private physicians. In essence, the availability of hospitalists would

106

free private physicians from the many responsibilities associated with hospitalizing patients and arranging coverage.

Unfortunately, the hospitalist concept is not without significant downside potential. For starters, the concept gives full control of hospitalizations to hospital administrators and health insurers, and threatens to interfere in the decision-making of physicians employed as hospitalists.

With hospitalists under their control, hospitals can better control the length of hospital stays, the drugs that are dispensed via the hospital formularies and the availability of in-patient testing, consultations and procedures. What's more, through the on-going processes of downsizing and downskilling, the hospitals can gain greater autonomy and effectively divorce the medical staffs that once played a prominent role in the policy-making of their institutions.

It is no coincidence the development of the hospitalist concept has paralleled the emergence of managed care in America. Consequently, a possible side effect of the management of patients by hospitalists could be the recruitment of hospitalized patients into managed care programs and the redirection of many of these patients away from private physicians who are not in managed care's good graces and into the waiting arms of physicians who are.

At best, the hospitalist concept is a two-edged sword. Whereas the availability of hospitalists can potentially improve the health care of many communities, that same availability can also work to the detriment of the medical profession by allowing outside forces to gain control over an increasing number of physician employees.

With this in mind, it would appear the best interest of patients and physicians would be served by allowing hospitalists and private physicians to work side-by-side in the same hospitals. Private physicians should be allowed to hospitalize their own patients and hospitalists allowed to manage unreferred patients or patients voluntarily referred to them by private physicians.

To this end, universal rules of conduct that govern the transfer of patients between private physicians and hospitalists should be formulated by the medical profession. Such rules should include prohibitions against the use of the hospital as a recruiting center for managed care programs or other health care providers.

What's more, the use of hospitalists or private physicians should not be turned into an "either-or" proposition by any hospital. Hospitals should be allowed to employ hospitalists, but not allowed to prohibit or limit the hospitalizations of patients by private physicians.

Similarly, health insurers should be permitted to reimburse patients for services rendered by hospitalists, but not allowed to deny or discount reimbursement for hospital services provided by private physicians. As in the case of hospitals, health insurers should not be allowed to discriminate against physicians in any manner.

To understand the various implications of the current hospitalist movement in the United States is to understand managed care works in strange and mysterious ways. To understand the workings of managed care is to understand why the lives of so many American physicians have become as shaky as a fiddler on the roof.

October, 1998

POINT OF SERVICE

Three young brothers celebrated the end of each work week by going to a local tavern and drinking a glass of beer. When two of the brothers moved away, the remaining brother decided to uphold the family tradition.

Each Friday after work, the young man would go to the same tavern and proudly announce that he wanted three beers - one for himself and one for each of his brothers. With time, the tavern's patrons looked forward to seeing their favorite bartender serving three beers at a time to the personable young man with strong family ties.

One Friday after work, the young man entered the tavern and requested two beers.

"I don't mean to pry," the bartender said, "but why only two beers? Did something happen to one of your brothers?"

"Oh, no," the young man replied. "My brothers are fine, but I've decided to give up drinking for Lent!"

Just as the young man decided to give up drinking, many Americans have decided to give up health care. Managed care is the reason and a phenomenon known as "Point of Service" is the latest variation on managed care's theme of health care rationing to patients and fee rationing to physicians.

For no other reason than to create the illusion it offers its patients freedom of choice, managed care has now created Point of Service contracts. As the name suggests, such contracts allow patients to obtain health care both within and outside the managed care network.

In theory, Point of Service almost sounds like the traditional American way of doing business. Unfortunately, the concept is an old-fashioned apple pie with more crust than fruit.

109

Admittedly, Point of Service allows managed care patients to choose their own health care providers, but this is where freedom of choice falters. Through a highly discriminatory fee schedule, managed care pays its own providers one fee and providers outside the network a drastically reduced fee, thereby burdening patients with excessive out-of-pocket expenses and conditioning them to obtain health care services exclusively from managed care providers.

If the word, "discriminatory," seems a bit harsh to describe Point of Service, consider a few of the more salient features of a typical Point of Service contract I recently reviewed. For starters, managed care patients with such contracts usually pay no deductibles for health care received within the managed care network, but typically pay a yearly deductible in the neighborhood of $250 for services obtained outside the network.

What's more, such patients can be charged stiff penalties for obtaining unauthorized services outside their network. A patient with a Point of Service contract, for example, can see a physician outside the network and have an MRI scheduled but, if the test is not pre-authorized by the patient's managed care organization, the patient can be held liable for the first $400 of the MRI's cost.

Many Point of Service programs pay 100% of those health care services rendered within the managed care network but only 70% of the managed care organization's approved charge for services rendered outside the network. If, for example, a physician who is not a member of the patient's managed care network charges the patient $50 for an intermediate office visit but the managed care organization's approved charge is only $40, the patient is reimbursed 70% 0f $40, or $28, and expected to pay the additional $22 for the service out-of-pocket.

Managed care patients with such Point of Service contracts are typically reimbursed 70% of the approved charges submitted by non-participating health care providers for: office services, in-patient services, surgery, anesthesiology, maternity care, radiological services, lab tests, allergy treatment, physical therapy, skilled nursing, home health care, hospice care, private nursing, durable medical equipment, chemotherapy, radiation therapy and dialysis. Such services usually have yearly monetary limits attached, and the patient is responsible for the difference between the actual charges and the managed care organization's payment.

At the very least, Point of Service contracts are unfair and discriminatory in nature. Such contracts place an unfair financial burden on patients who choose to obtain health care outside the managed care network, and give managed care providers an unfair advantage in the health care marketplace.

When financial burdens become too great for patients who obtain health care services outside the managed care network, they are forced back inside the network by default. When such patients re-enter the network, their former physicians lose patients, as well as income.

Betwixt and between the black and white of managed care is a gray area that is currently home to a vast number of patients who cannot go back to their private physicians because of an inability to pay for 30% of their health care, and who refuse to see managed care providers because of their previous experiences with health care rationing. As a result, these patients have rejected the entire American health care system and currently receive no medical care whatsoever.

This generally unrecognized phenomenon, of course, allows managed care to continue claiming it has effectively contained health care spending in America. If scads of managed care patients are unable to afford private physicians and unwilling to see managed care physicians, the end result is major league savings for the managed care organizations, not to mention the spurious statistics that allow such corporations to justify their continued existence.

Point of Service contracts are unfair to patients, discriminatory to the health care providers who do not participate in managed care and a direct violation of most labor laws and industry standards, both real and implied. What's more, Point of Service contracts are just a single connecting line away from the final point where American health care is heading - the point of no return!

May, 1998

RICHES TO RAGS

In a city known for its outstanding physicians, he was considered one of the best. For two decades, he nurtured the pediatric practice he founded and, by quiet example, helped his partners set new standards for the health care of children.

To watch him around frightened youngsters or apprehensive parents, you would never associate him with the big house in which he lived or the expensive car he drove. He had earned the right to act in a manner commensurate with his success, but he chose to act as a common man whose humility clearly overshadowed his trappings.

When managed care came to town, he had more than his fair share of misgivings. He knew that, if he refused to join a managed care network, many grateful families would keep their conventional health insurance or even pay cash to retain his professional services.

Like so many other truly great physicians, however, he cared more about people than money, and he was always trying to make life easier for those who entrusted him with their health and well being. Accordingly, he allowed the medical practice he had conceived and developed to become part of a managed care conglomerate that promised to facilitate health care delivery to his many patients.

It didn't take long for him to discover his patients had become managed care's patients and his style of practice worked only when it jibed with managed care's philosophies. It didn't take long for him to realize managed care was insidiously turning his medical practice into an assembly line.

Perhaps he had been too busy to read the growing number of horror stories about managed care in the medical literature. Perhaps he had been too trusting to carefully study the sections on gag orders, physician deselection and restrictive covenants in the legally-binding managed care contract he signed.

Regardless of the reason, this man of vision and foresight never saw managed care coming. He didn't realize how quickly riches could be shredded into rags.

When he complained about the deterioration of the medical practice he had founded twenty years earlier, his complaints fell on deaf ears. When he complained louder, his paychecks were stopped.

Feeling there was something inherently wrong with a physician being forced out his own medical practice, he hired the best lawyers money could buy. As his savings dwindled and he was no longer able to pay the mortgage on his beautiful home, he quickly discovered the futility of trying to personally finance a legal battle against a large corporation.

In a city known for its outstanding physicians, one of its finest now sits unemployed in a small rented townhouse. By order of their new employer, his former partners are being forced to disavow any knowledge of his whereabouts as they attempt to assimilate his many patients into their crowded practices.

It is tragic it took the loss of a medical practice to make this physician, and too many others like him, realize managed care's only motive is corporate profit. As a growing body of evidence continues to show, managed care's profit is, all too often, everyone else's loss.

February, 2001

APPLES AND ORANGES

The January 5, 2000 edition of the *Journal of the American Medical Association* contains a paper, entitled, *Primary Care Outcomes In Patients Treated By Nurse Practitioners Or Physicians*. The study's authors are affiliated with the Columbia University School of Nursing.

Claiming that "studies have suggested that the quality of primary care delivered by nurse practitioners is equal to that of physicians," the paper's authors set out "to compare outcomes for patients randomly assigned to nurse practitioners or physicians for primary care follow-up and ongoing care after an emergency department or urgent care visit." Their research was conducted at a primary care clinic of the Columbia-Presbyterian Medical Center in New York City, as well as 4 urban satellite clinics that "serve primarily families from the Dominican Republic who are eligible for Medicaid (and) are primarily immigrants (who) frequently change their residences (and) travel between New York and their country of origin."

In this study, 1,316 patients "who had no regular source of care and kept their initial primary care appointment" were screened from a group of 3,397 patients, and randomly assigned to either a physician (510 patients) or a nurse practitioner (806 patients). The patients who were enrolled in the study had a mean age of 46 years; 77% of the patients were female and 90% of the patients were Hispanic.

Patient satisfaction with their health care provider was measured by a 15-item questionnaire immediately and 6 months after the initial appointment. Patients were assisted with questionnaires and interviews by bilingual interpreters.

Health status, as measured by the "Medical Outcomes Study Short-Form 36," and physiologic test results were recorded 6 months after the initial appointment. The physiologic tests included measurements of blood pressure in hypertensives, hemoglobin A1C levels in diabetics and peak air flow measurements in asthmatics.

Finally, health services utilization was obtained from computer records for 1 year after the initial appointment. Outcome measures were compared according to the type of provider.

Although a number of the nurse practitioners who participated in the study were identified as faculty members at the Columbia-Presbyterian Medical Center, the research paper did not indicate the status of its participating physicians. Accordingly, one cannot establish if the study attempted to compare the performance of experienced nurse practitioners to physicians-in-training, board-certified physicians or an admixture of physicians with different levels of education, certification and professional experience.

With the exception of small differences in diastolic blood pressure measurements and the provider attribute dimension of patient satisfaction, patients randomly assigned to physicians and those assigned to nurse practitioners demonstrated no significant differences in health status at 6 months, diabetic or asthma test results at 6 months, health services utilization or other measures of patient satisfaction. As a result, the authors concluded that "in an ambulatory care situation in which patients were randomly assigned to either nurse practitioners or physicians and, where nurse practitioners had the same authority, responsibilities, productivity and administrative requirements, and patient population as primary care physicians, patients' outcomes were comparable."

This study's authors set out to prove the quality of primary care delivered by nurse practitioners is equal to that of physicians. What their study actually demonstrated is that a sample of predominantly female Hispanic immigrant patients appeared satisfied with the free short-term follow-up medical care they received, regardless of the professional status of their provider, and certain diseases can be treated by non-physicians.

To better understand what this study did and did not demonstrate, first consider the participants. Consider how the data might have changed if discriminating middle-class American citizens who didn't require the assistance of an interpreter, who truly understood the significant differences between physicians and nurse practitioners and who had to pay for their own health insurance were used instead of the original study participants.

Consider also how satisfaction levels and health services utilization might have changed if the patients were followed for 6 years instead of 6 months. Consider how these same parameters might have changed once previously diagnosed and stabilized medical conditions became more complicated over time and required more expert treatment.

While we're on the subject of medical conditions, consider the diseases that were monitored in this study. Interestingly, diabetes, asthma and hypertension are all diseases that are routinely treated by both physicians and nurse practitioners but, even more significantly, diseases that have proven amenable to self-monitoring and self-treatment by patients themselves.

Consider the staggering number of adult-onset and juvenile diabetics who monitor their own blood glucose levels and adjust their own insulin or oral hypoglycemic dosages for prolonged periods of time without medical assistance of any kind. Consider also the number of asthmatics who routinely adjust their own medications without the supervision of physicians or nurse practitioners.

Consider, too, the number of hypertensives who monitor their own blood pressures and adjust their diets, exercise levels and medications for extended periods of time without consulting medical personnel. With the proper instruction, many diabetics, asthmatics and hypertensives have learned how to effectively control their diseases with only minimal professional support.

In addition to using different participants and measuring outcomes, patient satisfaction and health services utilization over longer periods of time, this study would have been much more credible if more challenging clinical situations had been used to measure the quality of medical care rendered by nurse practitioners. By demonstrating their ability to successfully diagnose and treat a teenage girl with a fever of unknown origin, a middle-aged man with chest pain and an elderly patient experiencing an acute confusional episode, illnesses routinely handled by competent primary care physicians, nurse practitioners would move closer to confirming this study's hypothesis.

If there is an injustice associated with this study, it is that a severely flawed research paper was published in a widely-read and frequently-quoted medical journal, and is destined to be used as propaganda by those bent on creating the illusion that the quality of primary care delivered by nurse practitioners is equal to that of physicians. It is inevitable managed care greed mongers who stand to profit financially when greater numbers of physicians are replaced by nurse practitioners, politicians who see cheaper medical care as a means to a balanced budget and left-wing nurse practitioner groups that have lost sight of their role in our health care delivery system will be quoting and misquoting the study for many years to come.

If there is a fundamental design error in this study, it is that attempting to compare physicians and nurse practitioners is like trying to compare apples and oranges. What results is one lemon of a research paper.

March, 2000

PHYSICIAN-ENTREPRENEURS

A physician recently sent me an audiocassette to evaluate. The cassette briefly introduced a program that is currently seeking physician-entrepreneurs to help market the products and services of a large pharmaceutical company.

In all honesty, the cassette was worth a listen. Our medicine cabinets still have room for a low-cost, natural product that can effectively lower lipids and increase dietary fiber, and the cassette extolled the virtues of such a product in a convincing manner.

To introduce this product, as well as the entrepreneurship thereunto pertaining, the cassette presented the testimonies of a few dozen physicians. Each physician presented his or her curriculum vitae, personal experience with the various products of the sponsoring pharmaceutical company and reasons for deciding to join the company as an entrepreneur.

The vast majority of the physicians recorded on the cassette were able to present impressive credentials, as well as convincing accounts of their success with the products they were marketing. These same individuals were also able to convey a message that clearly expressed a desire and/or need to start developing some sort of life after medicine.

Once upon a time, people entered the medical profession for predictable reasons, not the least of which was financial security. If a single audiocassette is any indication, it would appear success in the medical profession can no longer be used as a constant in any equation dealing with fiscal certainty.

As I listened to the cassette, I heard a number of seemingly intelligent and apparently skilled physicians decrying managed care, the health insurance industry and government as the culprits who were interfering with their abilities to thrive professionally and financially in the health care marketplace. In many of their voices, I could hear a scientist who was becoming a businessman by necessity rather than choice.

Listening to the cassette, I heard thoughtful individuals talking about working too hard, not having enough time for themselves or their families and not being able to predict how the ongoing socialization of health care in America would affect their financial security. In their voices, I could hear the experience that comes with many years of arduous medical training trying to blend in with the uncertainty that follows a crash course in corporate marketing.

America may not have invented entrepreneurship, but it has certainly been the concept's greatest proponent. America is the land of the free and, to some extent, the freedom to engage in multiple professions simultaneously, the freedom to change professions in mid-stream and the freedom to profit from one's own ingenuity have been byproducts of the American birthright.

Speaking first-hand, I can attest to the fact that, without entrepreneurship, at least one individual whose essay you are currently reading would have never had the chance to leave the other side of the proverbial railroad tracks and work his way through college, a graduate program and medical school. Without entrepreneurship, this same individual would not have been able to spend the past 18 years practicing medicine and raising a family in the financial insecurity of rural America.

Being an entrepreneur-of-sorts has always been one of my defining characteristics. Fortunately, this propensity has never interfered with my passion for being a doctor.

When I finished listening to the audiocassette, I was impressed by the energy, enthusiasm and versatility of many of its speakers. Unfortunately, I was also bothered by the fact many of the speakers sounded capable of leaving the medical profession in a heartbeat if a more lucrative opportunity presented itself.

To be sure, there is room in the lives of most physicians for an entrepreneurial frolic. In fact, a profitable avocation can be a healthy diversion from a demanding medical practice.

Unfortunately, too many physicians are not looking at current business ventures for the sole purpose of augmenting their incomes. Instead, they are looking at such ventures as a way out of medicine.

For too many years, government and the health insurance industry conspired to socialize medicine in America. For too many years, too many physicians sat back and watched as crooked politicians and greedy industrialists stacked the legal deck in their own favor and used the law to systematically dissemble America's tried-and-true health care delivery system.

With time, medicine was turned into a mere job for too many physicians, and the medical workplace was turned into a veritable sweat shop. When a physician's ability to pay bills and provide for a family were finally threatened and when organized medicine was unwilling or unable to offer any relief or solutions, physicians started to critically reevaluate their profession.

Is it any wonder, then, so many physicians have become so dissatisfied with a profession they worked so long and so hard to enter? Is it any wonder so many physicians have begun to explore any avenue that might eventually lead to an exit from this place called Medicine?

If the leaders of organized medicine in the United States are not bothered by the exodus of young physicians from the medical profession, they should be. The loss of physicians due to unfavorable working conditions, widespread job dissatisfaction and threatened financial security is an insult to those who have been entrusted with the responsibility of safeguarding the practice of medicine in America.

Similarly, medicine's elder statesmen should also be concerned about physicians being forced to venture outside the medical profession to augment their incomes. Should highly intelligent and highly skilled individuals who have contributed a dozen or more years of their lives as well as personal fortunes to medical education be forced to sell nutritional supplements so their bills might be paid or their financial goals met?

Throughout medicine's illustrious history, many physicians have entered into various business ventures for the sake of investing. Today, however, many physicians are being forced to enter into business ventures out of financial necessity.

Throughout its history, physicians have left medicine for any of a number of valid reasons. Today, an alarming number of physicians are prematurely leaving the medical profession because of intolerable working conditions, financial uncertainty and medicine's disgraceful inability to represent, protect or aid its members.

If there was ever a day when American health care needed a new direction, today is that day. If there was ever a time when the medical profession needed to unionize, reorganize and plot a new direction for American health care, that time is now.

I hope the next audiocassette I receive invites me to become an entrepreneur in a new physicians' union, a new medical profession and a new health care delivery system. That's one business opportunity I won't pass up.

August, 1998

MARIJUANA

Other cultures know the substance by such names as dagga, ganja and kif. Americans commonly refer to it as grass, pot and weed.

Other cultures have been known to ingest the substance as a food condiment or beverage spice. Americans commonly smoke the substance in cigarettes called joints or doobies.

The substance is derived from the hemp plant, Cannabis sativa. Blessed by many and cursed by more, the substance, of course, is marijuana.

Known to the Chinese nearly three-thousand years before the time of Christ, marijuana has served mankind as both a medicine and an intoxicant. Although marijuana has been freely used by many different cultures throughout history, use of the drug has been prohibited in the United States for the past sixty years.

In addition to its effects as a sedative, intoxicant and hallucinogen, marijuana is also a potent anti-emetic, appetite stimulant and intraocular pressure reducer. Because of these latter effects, the Food and Drug Administration (FDA) approved marijuana's active component, tetrahydrocannabinol, for medical use in 1986.

Known as dronabinol, synthetic tetrahydrocannabinol is an oral preparation that is currently approved for use as an appetite stimulant in patients with the acquired immunodeficiency syndrome (AIDS) and an antiemetic in cancer patients receiving chemotherapy. The drug is also used to treat select patients with glaucoma.

Although many patients with AIDS, cancer and glaucoma appear to have benefited from dronabinol use, many other patients with the same afflictions claim dronabinol is a poor substitute for marijuana. In recent years, representatives of this latter group have lobbied to have marijuana legalized for medical use.

In the November, 1996 elections, residents of California and Arizona flocked to the polls to vote on measures that would legalize marijuana for medical use in their respective states. The measures passed in both states with 56% of the California voters and 65% of the Arizona voters approving the medical use of marijuana.

In recent weeks, federal officials have warned that, regardless of any new state laws, physicians who prescribe marijuana should be prepared to experience the unbridled wrath of the federal government. Such wrath, of course, would most likely be expressed as a suspension or revocation of the offending physician's federal license to prescribe drugs - a license controlled by the federal Drug Enforcement Administration (DEA).

The loss of a physician's DEA license quickly cascades into the loss of state medical licensure, the loss of malpractice insurance coverage, the loss of hospital admitting privileges, the loss of medical practice and assorted other undesirable consequences. Clearly, the loss of a physician's DEA license is nothing short of professional suicide.

Whether or not marijuana should be legalized for medical use is not a single question but a whole host of interrelated questions. To complicate matters, none of these questions come with easy answers.

The first question that must be asked relates to the legitimacy of the argument that marijuana cigarettes are more effective medicinally than the currently available dronabinol pills. Is marijuana a more effective appetite stimulant, anti-emetic and anti-glaucoma drug than dronabinol?

If marijuana is not clearly superior to dronabinol, the discussion ends here. If, on the other hand, marijuana could conceivably help patients with AIDS, cancer and glaucoma, the questions continue.

124

Assuming marijuana is a more valuable drug than dronabinol, the next question relates to the safety and practicality of marijuana use. Is marijuana a safe and practical drug for patients to use, pharmaceutical companies to manufacture, pharmacies to merchandise, medical personnel to dispense and the general public to handle?

To be sure, marijuana has a tremendous abuse potential and an impressive array of deleterious side effects. However, so do narcotics, tranquilizers, sleeping pills, diet pills and a whole host of other currently available drugs, as well as alcoholic beverages which can be easily obtained without a prescription.

If marijuana use is unsafe and impractical, further questioning is moot. If marijuana's risk-to-benefit ratio is acceptable, however, there are still other questions to be asked.

Assuming marijuana could be used safely and discriminately, the next question relates to the jurisdiction of state and federal governments in the approval of drug use. Do states have the authority to approve drugs for use by their residents or does that authority reside solely with the federal Food and Drug Administration?

States clearly have the right to self-govern but their right to determine which drugs their residents use appears to be an entirely different matter. If California and Arizona were allowed to authorize the medical use of marijuana in their states, a dangerous precedent might be set for other states to follow.

In the near future, other states might authorize the medical use of other controversial drugs. Patients would then be forced to chaotically travel from state to state to obtain drugs unavailable in their own locales.

Clearly, the regulation of drug use belongs at the national, rather than the state, level. This being the case, however, who should be holding the reigns of the federal Food and Drug Administration?

Should FDA policy makers be listening to politicians, representatives of the special interest groups or scientists? Should the drugs we use be determined by a political agenda or by the scientific method?

In my 48 years on this planet, I have never smoked marijuana and I have never advised anyone to use the drug. I do acknowledge, however, that marijuana does possess medicinal qualities that could benefit patients with various maladies, and such patients should not be deprived of drugs with clinically-proven efficacy.

Accordingly, it is my belief the medical use of marijuana should be thoroughly re-investigated by the FDA and the agency's ultimate decision should be respected by the medical community. To this end, however, the FDA should be guided by the research of scientists and the clinical experience of practicing physicians, rather than the popular sentiment of uninformed voters, the ultra-conservative tack of our Ivory Tower medical societies or the hidden agenda of a drug culture that purports to be laboring on behalf of the sick and dying.

Marijuana has been used by mankind for over five-thousand years - many times uneventfully and many times controversially. It would appear the time has come for a new culture to redefine how mankind can best coexist with Cannabis sativa.

To this end, one might ask - doobie or not doobie? That seems to be the question!

February, 1997

WHAT PATIENTS SHOULD KNOW BEFORE THEY JOIN A MEDICARE HMO

All across the nation, elderly and disabled patients are deciding whether or not to join a Medicare health maintenance organization (HMO). There are a number of facts these patients should consider before they venture into the uncertain world of managed care.

For starters, Medicare patients should realize managed care and traditional health care are not the same. With traditional health care, i.e., health care financed by Medicare and supplemental health insurance, Medicare patients can choose their own primary care physicians, specialists and hospitals.

They can receive diagnostic tests and procedures, consultations with specialists, and in-patient medical and surgical care anywhere in the United States. In an emergency, these patients can be taken to the nearest hospital emergency room for immediate treatment and, while on vacation, their medical care can be transferred to Medicare providers in 50 different states.

With managed care, i.e., Medicare HMOs, Medicare patients are limited in their choice of physicians and hospitals. They can select a primary care physician from a list of available HMO doctors, but much of their actual care may come from nurse practitioners or other ancillary personnel.

For routine or emergency care, these patients can only use hospitals that are a part of their HMO's immediate network. Similarly, they can only be referred to HMO diagnostic centers and HMO specialists.

Diagnostic tests and procedures, consultations with and treatment by specialists, surgery and hospitalizations must be pre-authorized by their HMO. Although Medicare HMOs may pay for short-term emergency care rendered to patients who are traveling, they do not pay for routine medical services obtained outside the HMO network.

Second, Medicare patients should understand HMOs stay profitable by rationing health care. Managed care corporations ration health care because less health care translates into more corporate profit, and more corporate profit translates into higher performance bonuses for executives, fatter retirement packages for corporate directors and greater earnings for investors.

Unfortunately, rationing health care, especially to elderly patients with chronic illnesses, means corners must be cut. Nurse practitioners must work above the level of their training and function as physicians, primary care physicians must work outside the area of their expertise and render the kind of medical and surgical care that was once only provided by specialists, and specialists must limit the number of diagnostic tests they order, procedures they perform and drugs they prescribe.

All this, of course, results in compromised health care. When health care is compromised, medical malpractice may result.

Third, Medicare patients should know federal loopholes currently protect HMOs against malpractice litigation. If, for example, an HMO physician fails to order a necessary diagnostic test on a patient because the test is not approved by the patient's HMO, diagnosis and treatment can be delayed, resulting in patient injury or death.

If such an incident leads to a malpractice suit, the physician may be held accountable, but the real culprit - the HMO, may not. This is because the federal Employee Retirement Income Security Act (ERISA) exempts health plans that can be offered as an employee-benefit from state law.

Insofar as medical malpractice is governed by state and not federal law, many HMOs currently appear to be untouchable in legal actions involving medical malpractice.

If the physician who failed to order the necessary test because of HMO interference is exonerated in court and the HMO cannot be sued, the injured patient or that patient's heirs, could walk away from court without compensation.

Fourth, Medicare patients should realize the majority of elderly patients with chronic illnesses who are treated in HMOs can be expected to experience a decline in physical health. In a study published in the October 2, 1996 edition of the *Journal of the American Medical Association*, a group of physicians reported the results of their study of 2,235 chronically-ill, elderly and poor patients who received medical treatment over a four-year period of time in HMOs located in Boston, Chicago and Los Angeles.

Two-thirds of these patients experienced perceptible declines in physical health during the relatively brief period of time in which the research was conducted. Insofar as this study is statistically valid, elderly patients with chronic illnesses need to know HMOs may be dangerous to their health.

Fifth, Medicare patients should understand they are currently being lured into HMOs by deceptive advertising. For example, Medicare HMOs are advertising "prescription benefits" as a part of HMO enrollment.

This, of course, is interpreted by many senior citizens to mean "free medications." In truth, most Medicare HMO drug plans involve an $8 to $10 co-payment per prescription and have a $500 yearly limit.

Additionally, Medicare HMOs dispense only those drugs that are contained in their formularies. This deprives HMO patients of the benefits of many valuable drugs that are currently on the market but which HMOs refuse to authorize for use by their patients.

Medicare HMOs are also advertising premiums that are lower than those paid monthly by Medicare patients for supplemental health insurance. In some cases, the HMOs are even advertising a waiver of premiums.

This is deceptive because HMOs are not informing patients that these premiums will be dramatically increased once Medicare HMO enrollment reaches a critical mass. In all likelihood, the Medicare HMO premiums will eventually exceed the monthly premiums that Medicare patients are currently paying for supplemental health insurance.

HMOs are further deceiving prospective clients by not informing them that Medicare patients who are currently receiving traditional health care are only paying an average of $600 a year more than patients who are enrolled in Medicare HMOs. This is significant because patients are entitled to know a mere $600 a year separates comprehensive health care from rationed health care.

Sixth, Medicare patients should know it is difficult to investigate an HMO. If, for example, a prospective client is interested in learning the number of Medicare patients or number of physicians that have left a particular HMO, such information is difficult to obtain.

In reality, it is difficult to obtain any information about an HMO. For example, it is difficult to obtain information concerning patient or physician complaints against an HMO; legal actions against an HMO or its physicians; the educational and professional backgrounds of an HMO's medical staff, executives and directors; an HMO's track record with federal quality assurance studies; or the manner in which an HMO chooses to spend its money.

This past October, the General Accounting Office released a report, entitled, *HCFA Should Release Data To Aid Consumers, Prompt Better HMO Performance*. Later this year, the Health Care Financing Administration (HCFA) plans to provide consumers and health care professionals with comparative data on the nation's Medicare HMOs.

Instead of sending such information directly to Medicare patients and physicians, however, the HCFA has decided to provide this information via the internet. Unless the federal government plans to provide Medicare patients

130

with personal computers and internet software in the near future, investigating an HMO will remain a difficult pursuit.

Seventh, Medicare patients should realize an ever-increasing number of patients and physicians are currently leaving Medicare HMOs. Elderly patients, who are literally fearing for their lives, and concerned physicians, who are no longer willing to practice medicine within the confines of health care rationing, are making a quick exodus from the land of managed care.

When physicians leave an HMO, their patients must re-establish medical care with a new physician. During this frequently difficult transition, continuity of medical care can be disrupted.

When Medicare patients leave an HMO, they must frequently find another physician outside the HMO and obtain supplemental health insurance. For elderly patients, both tasks can be formidable.

Finally, Medicare patients should understand their tax dollars helped create the most sophisticated health care delivery system in the history of the world. Their tax dollars also fund the very legislative and judicial processes that are allowing managed care to take over the health care industry and profit as medical services are rationed to the very people who paid for their development.

Insofar as the tax dollars of Medicare patients helped create our health care delivery system, Medicare patients should receive the best health care that America can offer rather than the least health care that America is required to provide. Insofar as the tax dollars of Medicare patients continue to feed, clothe and house our legislators, the immediate needs of millions of elderly tax payers deserve at least as much consideration as the long-term needs of the corporate profiteers.

There are many reasons why Medicare patients belong in traditional health care programs rather than HMOs and an equal number of reasons why physicians should encourage elderly patients to stay away from managed care.

Respect for human life clearly stands out as the most important reason.

January, 1997

JOCKS AND DOCS

Many American children grow up with the dream of one day becoming a professional athlete. This is true of children who grow up in poverty, children who are born to wealth, and the vast majority of kids who spend their childhood somewhere in between.

For those children who grow up in poverty, professional athletics has historically represented one of the only visible means of legally escaping from the entrapments of their low socio-economic class. Entertainment has represented another.

In America, we are fond of talking about education as a way for the poor to pick themselves up by their boot straps. Unfortunately, very few children who are raised in American ghettos ever get the chance to climb the academic ladder.

We are also fond of talking about the military as a means of upward social class mobility for impoverished Americans. As with education, an inordinately small percentage of children from poor families ever get the chance to attain high military rank.

With this in mind, it should probably be of no surprise that more than just an occasional teenage athlete, who learned about sports on a weed-infested field or a litter-strewn playground, would forego health and well-being, and even risk life itself to play professional sports. When these kids talk about their willingness to die for a chance to play in "the show," they mean what they say - literally.

Bob Dylan once wrote, "...when you ain't got nothin', you got nothin' to lose." No one understands this more than poor children.

But dreams are not the exclusive property of the poor, especially when the dreams concern stardom in professional sports. Regardless of their trappings, kids from middle and upper socio-economic classes also dream of becoming athletic superstars, and many commit themselves to doing whatever it takes to make their dreams come true.

The recent death of Reggie Lewis, an event that has been widely covered throughout the news media, clearly demonstrates that, to many, a dream can be larger than life itself. Following a syncopal episode this past spring, a team of twelve cardiologists concluded Lewis suffered from hypertrophic cardiomyopathy and his return to the rigors of professional basketball was not advisable.

Significantly, this team of cardiologists had been consulted by the Boston Celtics, who stood to lose a great deal of money if Lewis could no longer play professional basketball. Despite the admonitions of the team of cardiologists, Lewis sought two other medical opinions.

These additional evaluations resulted in the conclusions Lewis was suffering from vasovagal syncope, a treatable condition that did not have to interfere with his professional basketball career. Lewis chose to continue playing basketball and, a few days prior to the start of training camp, he suffered a fatal cardiac arrest while engaging in a light workout.

A few years prior to Lewis' death, Loyola Marymount star, Hank Gathers, also suffered a fatal cardiac arrest while playing in a nationally-televised college basketball game. Like Lewis, Gathers was also diagnosed as having hypertrophic cardiomyopathy.

According to multiple published reports, Gathers was under medical treatment for this condition at the time of his death and aware of the possible consequences of playing basketball with a serious cardiac disorder. The fact Gathers was headed to the pros may have altered that awareness.

Before Hank Gathers came into prominence, we saw Sugar Ray Leonard risk, if not life, at least eyesight, to return to the professional boxing ring following a serious eye injury. And before Sugar Ray, we saw Muhammad Ali attempt one comeback after another in spite of progressive neurological dysfunction.

The list goes on and on. And what about the many American athletes who continued playing professional sports following disabling injuries?

Our fathers talked about Pete Gray, who played major league baseball with only one arm, and Monty Stratton, who returned to pitch in the pros following the loss of a leg in a hunting accident. Someday, many of us will probably tell our grandchildren about Jim Abbott, who didn't allow the absence of one hand prevent him from pitching for the New York Yankees, and Bo Jackson, who didn't let an artificial hip stop him from hitting home runs for the Chicago White Sox.

For every athlete who has risked life and limb to gain athletic prominence, there have been untold numbers of physicians whose medical and surgical skills have enabled these athletes to get through another practice, another game and another season. In rundown high school locker rooms, ivy-covered university field houses and sophisticated stadium treatment salons, physicians have employed conventional, as well as unconventional, treatment modalities to prepare their athletes for competition.

The story of the small-town doctor who enabled a high school football star with a fractured arm to play in the championship game by devising an ingenious splint is an old one. The stories of university and team physicians keeping their athletes on their respective playing fields at all costs are even older.

By repeatedly anesthetizing painful joints, by treating dehydration at half-time with rapidly-infused intravenous solutions and by dangerously accelerating growth and healing processes with steroids, mega-vitamins, dietary supplements, drug therapy and experimental diets, many physicians have provided quick fixes for the complications of athletic competition. In doing so, they have frequently maintained the health of a team at the expense of its athletes.

Sports, at the university and professional levels, are big business. There's bucks and perks in this corner of the wide world of sports, but with the spoils come expectations.

Athletes are expected to play with pain and their docs are expected to show them how. Disease or no disease, athletes are expected to "be there," and their docs are expected to let them.

As the limelight of professional athletics intensifies, a greater number of athletes can be expected to take a greater number of chances to secure a larger slice of an ever-expanding pie. Worrying about life-threatening arrhythmias and disabling injuries will be delegated to physicians while the athletes concentrate on adding their names to the record books and amassing fortunes in the process.

As long as college and professional sports are regarded as big business, athletes can be expected to disregard their illnesses and injuries and seek out physicians who will authorize their continued participation in athletic competition. As long as there is human nature and a sufficient number of motivating factors, there will be physicians to provide such authorization.

Shortly after testing positive for the human immunodeficiency virus (HIV), Magic Johnson's participation in Olympic basketball competition was publicly endorsed by an official of the American Medical Association. HIV transmission through contact sports, such as soccer and boxing, had already been reported in the medical literature but Magic's unrestricted participation in the Olympics was still endorsed by a physician who represented the standard bearer of organized medicine.

As long as America continues to worship its sports heroes, physicians will be expected to help prepare athletes for their next trip through the limelight. As recent events in the sporting world have clearly shown, such medical preparation is becoming more demanding and more consequential.

Physicians who render medical care to athletes must be careful of the limelight. If you stare at it too long, you can go blind; if you get too close to it, you can get burnt!

September, 1993

CONGRESSIONAL PHONE CALL

It's Friday morning, 9 A.M. The peace of morning in the country is suddenly disturbed by the ringing of the phone.

Me: Hello.

Caller: I'm trying to find Doctor Ra-mockers.

Me: This is Doctor Re-may-kus.

Caller: Of course, Doctor Reee-maaay-kus. I'm calling from Congressman Garblegarble's office. The congressman would like you to hear a brief message.

Me: Well, actually, I'm busy watching a flock of geese flying overhead.

Caller: Super. Here's the congressman, and I'll take your comments after his message.

Recorded message: This is Congressman Garblegarble. As one of America's leading physicians, I know you're concerned about the deplorable state of health care in this great nation. So am I. Managed care is stealing your profits. Your bottom line is being hurt by slow Medicare payments. The list goes on and on. You have a business to run, but the federal government seems to think you would rather be working for free. Well, with your help, I plan to change all this. I know I can count on you to join me in my crusade for health care reform. Stay on the line and one of my assistants will tell you how you can help.

Caller: Doctor Ra-mockers, I'll take your comments now.

Me: That's Doctor Re-may-kus.

Caller: Oh, yes, of course.

Me: First of all, does your congressman know anything about me?

Caller: Well, I'm not quite sure.

Me: How does he know I'm one of America's leading physicians?

139

Caller: Well...

Me: Are you aware of the fact a popular web site has named 2 out of every 3 American physicians to its list of leading physicians?

Caller: Is that right?

Me: That doesn't leave very many physicians for its list of followers, does it?

Caller: Well...

Me: Who ever heard of an army that needed 2 officers to lead one soldier, or a group that had 2 leaders for every follower?

Caller: Gee, you're right.

Me: But I digress. Other than contributing money, what would your congressman like me to do?

Caller: Well, the congressman was hoping you could make a contribution.

Me: At the risk of sounding redundant, what else can I do?

Caller: I don't think you understand. The congressman wants to fight for you.

Me: How?

Caller: He wants to help you handle managed care.

Me: I'd say I'm handling managed care pretty well on my own.

Caller: You are?

Me: Let me ask you something. If a tree falls in the forest but there's no one there to hear it crash, is there sound?

Caller: I don't understand.

Me: I don't participate in managed care. Ergo, it doesn't affect me. If more physicians would just ignore managed care, it would probably go away by itself.

Caller: Well, what about Medicare and how your business is being affected by its slow payments?

Me: You mean my practice, don't you?

Caller: Why, yes, of course, your practice.

Me: Considering I was a Medicare provider when Medicare used to send payments to the patient rather than the physician and, when Medicare used to pay $15 for a house call, I'd say Medicare has been doing pretty well lately.

Caller: Yes, but doctors don't make house calls any more.

Me: Some of us do.

Caller: Doctor, it sounds like you have some interesting ideas, but Congressman Garblegarble really wants to reform health care.

Me: So, did the other congressmen who passed the Employee Retirement Income Security Act to protect managed care against malpractice litigation, and the Health Maintenance Organization Act to provide tax advantages to managed care organizations and the McCarran-Ferguson Act to provide managed care with exemptions from antitrust laws. So are the current congressmen who are passing legislation that will allow nurse practitioners to practice medicine independently as though a master's degree was the equivalent of a medical school education and residency training. By the way, do you belong to an HMO or go to a nurse practitioner for your health care?

Caller: No, I don't.

Me: Does the congressman?

Caller: No, he doesn't.

Me: I rest my case.

Caller: Doctor, the congressman really is committed to health care reform.

Me: Then, tell the congressmen to start getting physicians, rather than politicians, involved in the reform process. How can congressmen reform what they don't understand?

Caller: Well...

Me: Health care reform will only occur in America from within the medical profession itself. Doctors, and not congressmen, must be the ones to reform health care.

Caller: Then, what are the congressmen supposed to do?

Me: I listened to your congressman's message. Now, I'd like you to listen to a message I've received over the internet on multiple occasions during the past few months. I don't know if there's any validity to this message, but I'd like your opinion.

Caller: Fine.

Me: Here goes the message verbatim. "Can you identify this outfit? Its employees have the following statistics: 29 have been investigated for spousal abuse; 7 have been arrested for fraud; 19 have been accused of writing bad checks; 117 have bankrupted at least two businesses; 3 have been arrested for assault; 71 are unable to get a credit card because of bad credit; 14 have been arrested on drug-related charges; 8 have been arrested for shoplifting; 21 are current defendants in lawsuits; and in 1998 alone, 84 were stopped for drunk driving. If you haven't guessed, these employees are members of the United States Congress, the same group that perpetually cranks out hundreds of new laws designed to keep every other American in line."

Caller: I'm not sure I understand.

Me: I don't know if there's any truth in this message but, if there's any truth at all, maybe the time has come for Congress to start taking better care of its own problems and start allowing doctors to handle health care reform.

Caller: Doctor, I'm making a note of your concerns and I'll make sure the congressman receives the note as soon as possible. In the meantime, may I send you some literature from the congressman, as well as a pledge card for a tax-deductible contribution?

Me: No, thanks. I'm into the Paperwork Reduction Act in a big way. You can do something, though.

Caller: What's that?

Me: You can tell the congressman health care reform will probably occur in a non-election year.

Caller: Oh, alright, Doctor Re-may-kus. Thank you. I'll be sure to share your thoughts with the congressman.

Me: Thanks for calling.

My wife from the next room: Bern, who were you talking to on the phone?

Me: Regis Philbin. Congressman Garblegarble wants to be a millionaire, and he tried using me as a lifeline.

March, 2000

A STATE OF DISUNION

A beautiful song from a bygone era begins with the line, "They're writing songs of love - but not for me." For some reason, that line kept going through my head as I listened to President Clinton's recent State of the Union address.

On January 23, 1996, the President gave his annual progress report to the American people in a speech that lasted 62 minutes. During that period of time, he spliced together many different words, but never once did he use the words, "doctor", "physician" or "health care provider".

In his State of the Union address, the President talked about what Congress wanted to do with Medicare and what the states wanted to do with Medicaid. Never once did he suggest what the half-million American physicians, who provide health care to Medicare and Medicaid patients, wanted to do with these programs.

In his speech, President Clinton talked about unprecedented economic growth in America, low unemployment rates, low interest rates, record corporate profits and a staggering Dow Jones Industrial Average. Never once did he mention that the income of the average American physician declined in 1995.

In his address, the President talked about continued economic prosperity for most Americans. Never once did he mention that a 2.3% decrease in Medicare payments for primary care services, decreased physician reimbursement from other government-sponsored health insurance programs and decreased physicians' incomes directly attributable to increased participation in managed care programs portend further income losses for physicians in 1996.

On January 23rd, President Clinton predicted continued prosperity for all Americans minus one-half million hard-working, patriotic, tax-paying physicians. He revealed his plans to improve American business and industry, but never once did he reveal any plans for funding medical education, stopping the socialization of American medicine or putting an end to the malpractice epidemic.

In his recent address, our chief executive tried to convince Americans of the healthy state of our union. Instead, he unwittingly demonstrated the undeniable state of disunion that exists in America today.

Years from now, historians will look back on 1996 as a year when America was a nation divided against itself. Videotapes of the 1996 State of the Union address will provide ample evidence that such was the case.

Democrats loudly cheering in concert at the slightest oscillation of the President's voice while an army of visibly unimpressed Republicans watch with lifeless expressions bespeak disunion. Scornful stares by Republican congressmen in the direction of other G.O.P. congressmen who appeared to support a few of the President's ideas bespeak another kind of disunion.

As videotapes of the State of the Union address clearly show, there is a profound lack of unity in the political leadership of the United States. Unfortunately, this contagious disunity has filtered down through every strata of American society and adversely affected each component of contemporary America, including our medical profession.

Today, more than ever before, the American medical profession is a profession without leadership, without direction and without the ability to demand respect from society, its courts or its legislatures. What's more, it is a profession that has lost sight of its roots, its power and its responsibility.

Today, too many physicians have sold out their profession and become part of the problem rather than the solution. Consequently, the medical profession has become one that boasts more second-lieutenants than foot soldiers and, as such, one that is ill prepared to fight the important battles.

Silver-tongued politicians can talk about budgets, deficits and reforms until they start to exhibit facial cyanosis but, without national unity, their talk is rhetoric and their plans are meaningless. Our elected officials must start thinking independently and doing what's best for all Americans and not just those who are willing and able to demonstrate party loyalty.

Similarly, physicians can talk all they want about the economic woes and political strife that befall the medical profession but, without professional unity in the timeless tradition of the Hippocratic Oath, their talk will continue to fall on deaf ears. Physicians must reunite and fight until medicine's rightful place in society has been restored.

Many different teams of horses are currently harnessed to our great nation. Unfortunately, the teams that represent the various components of contemporary American society are all pulling in different directions.

This has left America with an illusion of sustainable progress and prosperity. When the dust finally settles, all that may be left is a country that is destined to stand still for too long a period of time.

All Americans, regardless of class, profession or political affiliation, must redirect all our horses in the same direction. If this is allowed to happen, America will once again move swiftly, powerfully and confidently in the direction Adams, Franklin and Jefferson once envisioned.

All of us who were fortunate enough to be born into the freedom that is America must give deeper thought to the concept of unity. When we start doing this, State of the Union addresses will once again become what the name implies.

February, 1996

CPR RECERTIFICATION

A three-year-old child recently died while having dental work performed under general anesthesia. In the two months following the child's death, the oral surgeon who administered the anesthesia has already been sued for malpractice, arrested for involuntary manslaughter and notified his licenses to perform dentistry and administer general anesthesia have been suspended.

The oral surgeon's accusers have argued he did not have the proper emergency equipment available when he administered general anesthesia to the child. They have also argued he performed cardiopulmonary resuscitation (CPR) on the child without a current CPR recertification card.

No one has formally accused the oral surgeon of not knowing how to perform CPR. However, his detractors have accused him of not being able to adequately document that he participated in a recent CPR recertification program.

In the early 1960's, Kouwenhoven, Jude and Knickerbocker introduced external chest compression as a technique to combat cardiac arrest. By the mid-1960's, the National Academy of Sciences was recommending health care professionals learn this technique according to standards that were being developed by the American Heart Association (AHA).

In 1973, the AHA revised its standards for CPR and introduced standards for advanced cardiac life support. By 1980, the AHA was able to publish a definitive and comprehensive resource on cardiopulmonary resuscitation and emergency cardiac care in the Journal of the American Medical Association.

The early 1980's saw American medical schools and hospitals starting to routinely offer CPR training to their students, residents and veteran physicians. With time, an increasing number of other health care professionals learned the technique and rapidly passed it on to the general public.

Today, millions of Americans have learned how to perform CPR. In fact, CPR certification has even become a prerequisite for graduation from many American high schools.

CPR is an easy technique to learn and a difficult technique to forget. It's like swimming or riding a bike - hard to forget once learned.

Still, the American Heart Association has chosen not to issue permanent CPR certificates. Instead, it has chosen to certify and recertify individuals for relatively brief periods of time.

Now, here's the rub.

Periodic CPR recertification is not a requirement of any state or federal licensing board, credentialing board, professional society, peer review organization or professional liability insurer. Periodic CPR recertification is required by hospitals and other employers of health care professionals as a condition of employment or membership, but CPR recertification of health care professionals engaged in private practice is not mandated by state or federal law.

Unfortunately, not everyone understands the law and, when things go wrong, a physician's failure to produce a current CPR recertification card can be made to sound like professional negligence of the highest degree. No one has ever demonstrated the need for or value of CPR recertification but, as long as some physicians recertify and others don't, the malpractice lawyers have an extra card to play in court.

So, why don't all physicians renew their CPR certification on a regular basis? Could it be a physician or other health care professional who has performed CPR on hundreds of patients may not feel the need to relearn a skill he or she has already mastered?

Could it be not every health care professional has convenient access to CPR training sessions? Could it be many health care professionals have serious reservations about the safety of going mouth-to-mouth with a manikin that harbors viruses, bacteria and countless other disease-producing microorganisms?

For these and other valid reasons, many physicians and other health care professionals choose not to renew their CPR certification on a regular basis. As a result, these professionals run the risk of having their abilities challenged by opportunistic laymen who better understand how to create confusion than to respond to medical crises.

Each health care profession would benefit by having all its members periodically recertified in CPR. However, there's got to be a better way to accomplish this goal than by having health care professionals lining up for the chance to kiss Resusci Anne.

Insofar as health care professionals would benefit more by reviewing the theory behind CPR than by practicing chest compressions on a dummy, they could become recertified in CPR on a regular basis as a part of their state professional license renewal procedure. With their license renewal application, physicians and other health care professionals could be sent the same pamphlet the American Heart Association currently uses to teach CPR.

Following a review of the various CPR techniques, the health care professional could complete the same short written test that the AHA currently administers to individuals who are attempting to become certified in CPR for the first time. A passing score on the test would serve as a prerequisite to state license renewal and ensure CPR recertification.

Having performed CPR on hundreds of patients, I am well aware the technique involves more than just being able to locate a sternum and knowing when to exhale. Realistically, though, CPR doesn't require nearly as much

151

skill as many of the other medical and surgical procedures most physicians routinely perform with much greater frequency.

If physicians and other health care professionals can be trusted to perform difficult and potentially dangerous procedures on patients without periodic recertification, they can certainly be trusted to perform relatively simple procedures like CPR in a similar manner. Expecting physicians to repeatedly demonstrate their ability to perform CPR on a manikin is unreasonable and unnecessary, but asking physicians to periodically review the theory behind CPR in conjunction with state license renewal appears to be a workable compromise.

If an average American witnessed a cardiopulmonary arrest and attempted to perform CPR on the victim, even the most skeptical onlooker would call him a hero. What's more, no one would ask to see his CPR recertification card.

September, 1996

A QUESTION UNASKED

A prospective client asked a lawyer how much he charged for his legal services.

"I charge $1,000 for 3 questions," the lawyer replied.

"Isn't that a bit much?" the client asked.

"Yes, it is," the lawyer answered. "Now, what's your third question?"

Unlike the attorney in this story, physicians have never caught on to the idea of charging by the question. Insofar as physicians ask more than their fair share of questions with each patient encounter, fee-for-question medicine remains an impractical concept.

Although physicians ask many germane questions, there is one question too many practitioners still fail to ask their elderly patients on a routine basis. The question concerns a patient's wish for cardio-pulmonary resuscitation or extended life support in the event of an unexpected accident or illness.

Studies have shown health care providers are generally unaware of the resuscitation and life support wishes of their elderly patients. The same studies have shown many family members and personal caregivers are also guilty of the same oversight with their parents, close relatives and elderly patients entrusted to their care.

Unfortunately, the unexpected does happen - and usually at inopportune times. Apparently healthy elderly patients do experience strokes while watching television, cardiac arrests while undergoing elective surgery and various levels of brain damage when unexpectedly involved in serious accidents.

The unexpected does happen. In too many cases, however, families and health care providers are unprepared for that which follows the unexpected.

In too many situations, family members and medical personnel find themselves debating whether or not to resuscitate or provide extended life support to an elderly patient who has been rendered unconscious by a life-threatening accident or medical catastrophe. Invariably, the decision-makers ask each other about the patient's wishes but, all too often, such wishes are unknown to everyone except the unconscious patient.

As a result, lengthy, elaborate and expensive extended life support is provided to a high percentage of comatose patients by default. In many of these cases, the resuscitations, defibrillations and use of respirators and other life support modalities are provided against the express but, previously unspoken, wishes of the patient.

To be or not to be resuscitated is a question every person must ask him or herself. It is also a question that must be answered in the presence of the health care professionals who might be expected to resuscitate the patient or issue the order that obviates resuscitation and other extended life support measures.

Almost as important as asking the question about resuscitation and life support is the time and place the question is asked. Asking a frightened octogenarian who is moments away from elective cataract surgery if she would like to be resuscitated in the event of an adverse reaction to anesthesia or some other unexpected cardio-pulmonary mishap is a good example of bad timing.

Instead of asking an elderly patient about their wishes for resuscitation and life support during an emergency, crisis or anxious moment, the question should be asked at a calmer time when a life-threatening catastrophe does not appear to be imminent. A routine office visit is a good time to discuss a patient's wishes for future emergency care, and the office note is a good repository for the patient's response.

Most legal authorities would argue duly-processed living wills or advance directives are the proper way for a patient to express their wishes for or against resuscitation and extended life support. Unfortunately, time, effort and expense dissuade many elderly patients from creating such legal documents, while a lack of awareness of the importance or availability of such documentation prevents many other elderly patients from doing the same.

Although physicians should encourage their elderly patients to create a living will, advance directive or analogous document, the message remains more important than the media. Documenting the patient's wishes for or against resuscitation and extended life support in the office notes may not be as good as a notarized living will, but it is still a valuable record of the patient's wishes, pending more formal documentation.

Many health care professionals and family members who feel uncomfortable discussing death and dying with their patients or relatives would be surprised at the ease and candor with which most elderly patients discuss the subject. The vast majority of these patients want to be involved in the decision-making processes that affect their future health care, and they want the opportunity to share their thoughts, beliefs and wishes with their doctors and loved ones.

For any of a multitude of reasons, many elderly patients do not want to be resuscitated or have their lives mechanically sustained in the event of a serious accident or life-threatening illness. They'll tell you – if you ask them!

June, 1998

A CONSPIRACY THEORY

In light of the many conspiracies that have occurred in America in recent years, as well as Hollywood's current proclivity for making films about larger-than-life characters who conspire with one another, it has become suddenly mundane, if not unfashionable, to label anything a conspiracy. "Must everything in America be explained on the basis of some conspiracy?" a skeptic recently asked.

Everything in America doesn't have to be explained on the basis of some conspiracy, but to deny managed care is the result of a deep-seeded, far-reaching and well-planned conspiracy between business and government is to deny the obvious. How, other than through conspiracy, could laws be constructed to protect laymen who profit excessively from the rationing of health care and the systematic dissembling of the American medical profession?

If this is not the case and if managed care is the inevitable consequence of a health care delivery system gone awry rather than a conspiracy that allows businessmen and politicians to profit from the socialization of medicine in America, there should be answers to the many questions that still surround managed care. For starters, if managed care is not a conspiracy, why has the American medical profession been excluded from the development and implementation of health care policy in the United States?

Why did Hillary Clinton's federal health care task force utilize a secret war room to hold closed sessions in which private documents concerning American health care were generated? Why did this same federal health care task force refuse to cooperate with the District Court of the District of Columbia and turn over task force payroll records, minutes of meetings, agendas and affiliations of task force members, and open a public reading room where such records and documents could be inspected?

If managed care is not a conspiracy, why have the provisions of the Hill-Burton Act been disregarded? Why did the government allow 700 American hospitals to close between 1980 and 1990 when the Hill-Burton Act specifically calls for each state to maintain 5 hospital beds per 1,000 population?

Why are so many Americans still being denied hospitalization when the Hill-Burton Act mandates that hospital beds be made available to patients regardless of their ability to pay? If managed care is not a conspiracy, why do most large cities now have 3.5 hospital beds available per 1,000 population rather than the 5 beds mandated by the Hill-Burton Act?

Why are plans being made to decrease this number to 1.5 hospital beds by the end of the century? Why are plans also being made to further downsize hospital departments involved in acute care and further downskill hospital nursing and technical staffs?

If managed care is not a conspiracy, why have the states that have closed the greatest number of hospital beds also generated the largest health maintenance organization (HMO) enrollments? Why have states like Massachusetts and Illinois, which have large numbers of teaching hospitals, closed nearly one-quarter of their hospital beds?

Why has a state like New York, which has witnessed the closing of 75 hospitals in New York City alone in the past 30 years, agreed to participate in a program that will pay its teaching hospitals not to teach residents? If managed care is not a conspiracy, why is the government forcing Americans to currently sacrifice the benefits of the most sophisticated health care delivery system in the history of the world so the United States can finally balance its budget sometime next century?

Why is the United States ignoring its option to immediately erase its national debt by selling a mere fraction of its 60 trillion dollars' worth of assets, such as the land occupied by closed military bases, vacant military buildings and mothballed military equipment? Why, if the federal government is so concerned about balancing the budget, did it abandon consideration of a national health insurance program that would provide comprehensive health care to every American and, at the same time, spend 3% less of our gross national product on health care, 20% less per capita on health care and only 17% of the amount currently being spent on the administration of government-sponsored health care programs?

If managed care is not a conspiracy, why did the federal government create the Employee Retirement Income Security Act (ERISA) to protect HMOs against malpractice litigation? Why did it take so long for government to prohibit managed care organizations from imposing gag orders on physicians?

Why have only 8 states passed laws requiring managed care programs to provide written explanations to deselected physicians, and only 6 states passed laws requiring managed care organizations to provide deselected physicians with a formal appeals process? If managed care is not a conspiracy, why is the government ignoring scientific studies that have demonstrated 2 out of 3 chronically ill or disabled patients can expect a decline in physical health if their health care is turned over to a managed care organization?

Why is the government ignoring scientific studies that have demonstrated Medicare HMOs do not save money? Why is the government conveniently disregarding the fact there will be twice as many senior citizens as teenagers in the United States by the year 2005, a projected quadrupling of the incidence of Alzheimer's Disease in the United States within the next 40 years, and many other statistical realities that portend a need for an expanded, rather than retrenched, health care delivery system?

If managed care is not a conspiracy, why are managed care organizations being allowed to raise premiums and cut back on services so their yearly 20-30% profitability can be ensured? Why are managed care executives being allowed to collect yearly multi-million-dollar performance bonuses while patients are being deprived of necessary medical care, surgery, diagnostic testing, consultations and hospitalizations?

Why are managed care organizations being allowed to trim their budgets by using physician extenders in situations that require the training and experience of physicians? If managed care is not a conspiracy, why are managed care patients prohibited from crossing state lines to receive health care?

Why are employers being allowed to enroll their workers in health care programs that reimburse 100% of health care services obtained through managed care but only 70% of services obtained through conventional health care? Why is the federal government still threatening to prosecute physicians who fail or refuse to collect co-payments and deductibles from their Medicare patients, but allowing elderly patients to become enrolled in Medicare HMOs that do not charge co-payments or deductibles?

While you're trying to answer these questions, I'll be at the movies with my family. We're going to see *Conspiracy Theory*!

December, 1997

THE MEDICINE PROGRAM

As government and insurers continue to talk about providing prescription drug benefits to Americans, millions of chronically ill patients continue to face the existing hardship of finding ways to pay for their next supply of medications. This hardship is unnecessary.

The Medicine Program is a program that provides free prescription drugs to needy patients by matching the specific drug requirements of the patients with the availability of such medications through the patient assistance programs of the drug manufacturers. For the past year I have helped my needy patients obtain free prescription drugs through *The Medicine Program*, and I am happy to report this program really works.

For the past six years, *The Medicine Program* has provided free prescription drugs to low-income patients who do not qualify for government assistance, do not have insurance coverage for prescription drugs and cannot afford to buy such medications, as well as to middle-income patients who require expensive drugs for the treatment of such conditions as cancer, the acquired immunodeficiency syndrome (AIDS) or organ transplant rejection. Most of *The Medicine Program's* clients are retired, disabled or in a class of patients whose family incomes range from below the current poverty level to $50,000 yearly.

To request free prescription drugs, a patient first obtains an application from *The Medicine Program* at P.O. Box 515, Doniphan, Missouri 63935-0515, by phone at (573) 996-7300, or at their internet site, www.themedicineprogram.com. After they provide their name, address, phone number, current prescription drugs, and name and address of their physician, the patient returns the application with a one-time payment of $5 for each prescription drug requested.

After the application is processed, the patient receives a packet from *The Medicine Program* that contains request forms from the manufacturers of the requested drugs. These forms are generally short, straightforward and easy to complete.

Most of the request forms require a physician's signature and prescriptions for the drugs being requested. Once the forms are completed and the patient has kept copies with which to request future prescription refills, the forms are mailed or faxed from the physician's office to the drug companies.

If approved, most drug companies send a free three-month supply of the medications to the patient or physician within two to three weeks. Some companies send larger supplies of drugs or vouchers that can be redeemed by the patient at most pharmacies.

Each drug company has its own set of patient assistance criteria and each company is responsible for approving the requests for its own drugs. Therefore, a patient who requests a number of different prescription drugs through The Medicine Program may only qualify for or receive drugs from a percentage of the companies.

If a patient is determined ineligible and receives no free drugs through *The Medicine Program*, he or she is entitled to a full refund of the application fee. *The Medicine Program*, which continues to be endorsed by a growing number of government and social services programs, currently refunds 9% of fees to ineligible patients.

I have acquainted many patients with *The Medicine Program*, and each patient continues to receive free prescription drugs on a regular basis. *The Medicine Program* really works, and is an effective way for physicians to ease the financial hardship of their deserving patients.

September, 2001

SAVING MEDICARE

Following an exemplary life, an elderly gentleman died and went to heaven. When he was greeted at the Pearly Gates by Saint Peter, he was asked if there was anything he cared to see.

"This might sound strange," heaven's newest inhabitant told Saint Peter, "but before I spend eternity marveling at the wonders of heaven, I would really like to see what hell looks like."

Assuring the gentleman his request was not that uncommon, Saint Peter pointed to a window from which hell could be observed. A few minutes later, the old man returned with an astonished look on his face.

"Hell is nothing like I expected," the gentleman confessed. "I thought it would be all fire and brimstone, but all it looks like is a big, ice-covered canyon."

"Yeah, that happens every so often," Saint Peter replied. "It usually means someone in Washington just had an intelligent idea!"

A government official's intelligent idea might not be enough to make hell freeze over, but our government's latest attempts at saving the Medicare program make one seriously question the foresight, as well as motives, of those entrusted with the program's care. Admittedly, Medicare has its fair share of problems, but the program really isn't that hard to fix, maintain or preserve.

In recent months, Medicare has been working on a practice expense plan that would change the way Medicare providers are reimbursed. Of little surprise to no one except Medicare officials, such a plan has been very difficult to formulate.

For starters, any new practice expense plan by Medicare must be formulated in terms of the current resource-based relative value scale (RBRVS) that has

163

already undergone more perceptible changes than a fashion designer's mood ring. Years ago, Medicare handed expectant physicians the RBRVS with a promise of substantially higher fees for primary care services - a promise, of course, that has never been kept.

Using the RBRVS as a variable constant, Medicare officials have attempted to add a number of other variables to their new formula. These variables include reimbursements based on the actual amount of work a physician performs, practice expenses and the cost of malpractice insurance.

With the arrival of socialized medicine (a.k.a. managed care) in America, the majority of physicians have been working harder. Practices expenses, however, have varied greatly among physicians as have malpractice insurance premiums.

Many physicians, for example, have sold their practices to medical conglomerates, thereby significantly reducing their practice expenses, while other physicians, in their attempts to compete with the conglomerates and managed care corporations, have experienced greater professional expenditures. Similarly, physicians in many states have experienced decreases in malpractice insurance premiums due to a resurgence of competition in the malpractice insurance industry while physicians in states like Pennsylvania have experienced dramatic increases in malpractice insurance premiums because of the near-depletion of state catastrophe loss funds.

Medicare's archaic profile system notwithstanding, the formulation of a practice expense plan has been hindered by wide variations in practice expenses and malpractice insurance premiums. Throw Medicare's behavior offset into the formula, as well as the pending multi-billion-dollar government funding cuts to Medicare, and the formulation of a workable practice expense plan becomes a task even Einstein might have found too challenging.

164

The so-called behavior offset is a coefficient thrown into any equation dealing with Medicare reimbursement to physicians. It is based on the controversial theory that physicians will overutilize and overbill services to Medicare beneficiaries in an attempt to recoup anticipated financial losses brought about by cuts in Medicare reimbursement.

The bottom line here is Medicare is once again spending millions of taxpayers' dollars to concoct another in a long line of magical formulas by which Medicare providers can be reimbursed. Unfortunately, such a formula is, has always been, and will always be unnecessary.

Medicare doesn't need a new formula to guarantee its immediate or future solvency. All it needs is a quick tune-up and a new sense of direction.

For example, Medicare could save tons of money by simplifying its billing codes. Physicians don't need five different ways to bill an office visit, nor do they need more than one billing code for most surgical procedures.

By simplifying its billing codes and paying a fair price for the remaining services, Medicare could save a bundle. What's more, with simplified billing codes, Medicare could eliminate the need for its profligate research and phony audits, thereby saving even more money.

Medicare currently allows physicians to bill for office visits at five separate price levels and then spends millions of dollars yearly attempting to recoup money from physicians through audits. If Medicare only provided physicians with one fair price for an office visit, it would save enormous sums of money by curbing overcharges and other substantial sums of money by obviating its expensive auditing programs.

While it's waiting for such internal changes to take effect, Medicare could guarantee its immediate solvency by taking the advice of Senator Daniel Patrick Moynihan. The long-time Medicare proponent has previously suggested Medicare could be immediately saved by simply withholding one dollar from every social security check.

Along the same lines, the future solvency of the Medicare program could be ensured by taxing cigarettes and alcoholic beverages, and earmarking such taxes for future Medicare use. Just as those who are currently benefiting from Medicare could contribute to the program through social security deductions, those who will probably require greater amounts of medical care in the future, i.e., smokers and heavy alcohol users, could ensure Medicare's future solvency by paying taxes on the tobacco and alcohol they currently consume.

Saving Medicare is not as difficult as the politicians would have us believe. It just requires a fundamental understanding of the problem at hand and a little imagination.

Medicare officials can conveniently disregard such advice and labor until they turn blue in the face, but an elaborate practice expense plan will not survive the growing needs of Medicare's beneficiaries or providers. In fact, such a plan has about as much chance of surviving as a snowball in the place that freezes over whenever someone in Washington has an intelligent idea.

March, 1997

ALLOWING DOCTORS TO DECIDE

Recently, a rooftop party was held high atop a Manhattan skyscraper. Midway through the soiree, two inebriated party-goers made their way to the roof's edge.

"I think I'll jump off the roof and ride the air currents back up to the top," the first man said, handing his glass to a befuddled drinking partner.

Before his companion could react, the first man jumped off the skyscraper, fell half-way to the street and then gently floated back to the rooftop.

"Try it," he exclaimed, as he returned to the roof and retrieved his drink from his dumbfounded friend. "There's nothing more exhilarating than riding the powerful convection currents that swirl between these tall buildings."

After he finished his drink and briefly considered the encouraging words of his companion, the second man jumped off the building and fell straight to the pavement. As he fell, his former drinking partner smiled and raised his glass as if to propose a toast.

Watching the entire episode from a clear vantage point, another party-goer shook his head in disbelief.

"You know," the observer said to his date, "when he gets a few drinks in him, that Superman can be a real jerk!"

On November 8, 1999, one of America's largest managed care organizations (MCOs) announced it was eliminating its pre-certification requirement for many diagnostic tests, hospitalizations and surgeries, and effectively allowing physicians to have the final say in their patients' care. Although it retained its pre-certification requirement for certain procedures rendered within its own network and all treatment rendered by physicians or hospitals outside its network, the MCO announced it would stop many of the unnecessary hassles and delays associated with obtaining prior authorization.

Although the nation's second largest health insurer stated it was modifying its current pre-certification process to help eliminate "public ill will toward managed care" and to "restore the joy and art to practicing medicine for physicians," it also admitted the pre-certification process was costing more money than it was saving. In a recent experiment in which the prior authorization requirement was waived, the MCO was able to cut medical costs by 8% and hospital days by 9%.

When I heard the MCO's recent announcement, I immediately thought about the Superman story. What the announcement and story have in common is the implied admonition that things aren't always the way they seem.

It's true the MCO has formally acknowledged medical decisions should be made by physicians, but most insurers ultimately allow physicians to make their own decisions anyway. By adopting its new policy, the MCO will still be allowing physicians to make their own decisions - only sooner.

By eliminating pre-certification and the need to employ an army of pre-certification reviewers, the MCO will also be saving in excess of $100 million yearly. In an age of corporate bottom lines and inconsistent managed care earnings for stockholders, this retrenchment is no mere afterthought.

It's also true the MCO has made a concerted effort to project a new, user-friendly image by allowing patients and physicians to interact with reduced administrative interference. At a time when many employers and patients are choosing their health plans for next year and when many physicians are deciding which managed care organizations to join and which to drop, however, this makeover may be more rooted in the principles of shrewd marketing than philosophical enlightenment.

By creating a precedent that other managed care organizations will be forced to follow, the MCO also sends a loud and clear message to a Congress that has yet to enact into law the Norwood-Dingell Bill, or so-called "Patients' Bill Of Rights." The MCO's message is Congress need not legislate reforms for an industry that finally appears capable of reforming itself.

It's true the MCO has ceremoniously returned the final word in medical decision-making back to its physicians but, with a single public affirmation, the insurer has dramatically limited its exposure and liability to future malpractice litigation. With more states considering legislation that would allow patients to sue MCOs, the purveyors of managed care had to think of some way to stop the malpractice buck from traveling past physicians.

When the MCO publicly granted its physicians the right to make final decisions, it also returned the responsibilities that accompany that right to its doctors. Prominent among these responsibilities is that which requires an individual to accept any and all legal, professional and financial consequences of his or her actions, mistakes and maloccurrences.

However, when the MCO publicly granted its physicians the right to make final decisions, it maintained its own right to closely monitor the decisions of its physicians and review such decisions in audits and deselection proceedings. By giving its physicians more freedom to make their own final decisions, the MCO has also made its physicians more accountable, more vulnerable and more expendable.

At face value, the MCO's recent announcement appears to be a significant step forward for managed care, but the insurer has probably gained much more than it has relinquished, and physicians probably haven't gained as much as they originally thought. After all, things aren't always the way they seem.

So, think twice the next time Superman encourages you to jump off a rooftop. He may convince you the fall doesn't hurt - but forget to mention the sudden stop!

December, 1999

NATIONAL HEALTH INSURANCE

Yet another national health insurance bill has reached the floor of Congress. Introduced by Rep. Marty Russo, an Illinois Democrat, the latest plan would be funded through taxes and cover physicians' services, hospitalizations, preventive care, long-term care, mental health care, dental care and prescription drugs, all without co-payments or deductibles.

Thus far, the ambitious program has garnered the endorsement of various labor unions, including: the United Auto Workers; American Federation of State, County and Municipal Employees; American Postal Workers Union; International Ladies' Garment Workers Union; Amalgamated Clothing and Textile Workers Union; International Association of Machinists and Aerospace Workers; Oil, Chemical and Atomic Workers International; and Communications Workers of America. Since 50% of American corporate profits are consumed yearly in health care and 75% of American labor disputes and strikes are over health care benefits, the endorsement of national health insurance by organized labor should come as no surprise.

The willingness of Congress to once again listen to talk of national health insurance should come as no surprise either since the government-sponsored health care programs are in the process of self-destructing and the private insurance sector has been set into a tail spin by health care costs that continue to rise twice as fast as inflation. More and more people are starting to talk about national health insurance and more and more people are starting to listen to such talk.

The big question that still remains is whether or not a national health insurance program could be structured in such a way as to win the endorsement of the medical profession. Although the smart money would be betting against Medicine's unequivocal endorsement of any national health insurance program, the truth remains our current health care delivery system is not working and Americans are growing tired of spending more money for less health care.

When all the variables are plugged into the equation, it would appear national health insurance will one day become a fait accompli in the United States – possibly as early as the end of the century. It would also appear Medicine's latest challenge becomes the structuring of a national health insurance program that will benefit the medical profession as much as it will the rest of society.

National health insurance could work in the United States if such a program had the following characteristics:

1.) Program participation was optional for both physicians and patients. A successful national health insurance program would have to provide physicians with the freedom of either participating in the program or seeking reimbursement directly from patients or insurance companies. Similarly, such a program would have to allow patients the freedom of choosing a physician who didn't participate in the national health insurance program. In many ways, a successful national health insurance program would be similar to our public school system. Just as Americans are guaranteed a "free" public school education but can choose a private education at their own expense, Americans would also be guaranteed "free" medical services through the national health insurance program but would be able to obtain private medical care at their own expense.

2.) The program reimbursed physicians on a fee-for-service basis, the starting fees were in line with current levels of reimbursement at the time of program inception and plans were made to increase reimbursement for each service yearly using a federal "cost of living" index.

3.) The program provided physicians with the means for easy billing, rapid payment and hassle-free program participation. This could be accomplished by initiating a credit card format for billing, processing bills rapidly and laying to rest the erroneous, but popular, assumption that insurance fraud is the raison d'etre of every American physician. A successful national health insurance program would not waste money on frivolous utilization reviews and physician audits but would reserve such investigation for flagrant abnormalities in utilization and billing. Physicians or patients who were found guilty of program abuse could be denied future participation in the program.

4.) The program was financed by the federal government but run by an independent organization. In essence, a national health insurance corporation would act as an independent contractor of the federal government. For a national health insurance program to be successful, it would have to be run with administrative costs taking less than 2% of every health care dollar as opposed to the federal government's current 12%. For such a program to be successful, it would have to be run by physicians and businessmen and not by bureaucrats.

5.) The program provided its participating physicians with malpractice insurance, as well as a means of settling malpractice suits through arbitration. Insofar as the national health insurance program would be federally funded, any legal action against one of the program's participating physicians would also be an action against the federal government. This being the case, such actions could be settled through an arbitration board of the national health insurance program rather than the traditional court system. For any national health insurance program to be successful, dramatic new ways of handling this nation's malpractice epidemic would have to be devised. By taking malpractice out of the courtroom and moving it into arbitration, our $30 billion annual outlay in malpractice settlements would be dramatically reduced as would our

173

$30 billion annual outlay in unnecessary defensive medicine practices. Providing physicians with malpractice insurance and an equitable means of handling malpractice suits would help offset lost income by physicians, help insure physician participation in the national health insurance program and allow the medical profession and the federal government to labor together in good faith.

The question of national health insurance in the United States has become more a matter of "when" than "if." It would appear the time has come for all of us to gather our collective genius and create the kind of health care delivery system that will benefit both patients and physicians alike. If we don't, the federal government is apt to create another federal health care program that is sure to benefit no one but itself.

August, 1991

A MORE PERFECT UNION

It was once said what America needed was a good 5-cent cigar. That was many years ago, however, and America's needs have grown much more complex.

One of America's most pressing needs is health care reform. Unfortunately, such reform requires leadership, and no one seems willing to take the lead.

None of our presidential candidates seem capable of leading America toward the type of health care system it needs, and our Congress considers health care reform a conflict of interest. Most congressmen might appear to have IQs that are lower than their body temperatures, but they are smart enough to realize the special interest groups that are doling out the political action contributions are bent on keeping our current health care system in a state of chronic disarray.

Although every sector of America will ultimately need to participate in true and lasting health care reform, it is becoming more apparent the lead in health care reform will have to be taken by the medical profession. Unfortunately, the medical profession is ill prepared to take such a lead at the present time.

Before the medical profession can initiate serious health care reform, it must first develop a new sense of internal solidarity, as well as a mechanism for handling problems in a unified manner. This is why the time has come for everyone in the medical profession to seriously consider forming a union.

By "union," I am not referring to a medical society, some other American Medical Association (AMA) "wannabe" or some organization that would employ heavy-handed tactics to affect change. Instead, I am referring to an organization that would, through collective bargaining, provide American physicians with favorable working conditions and, in doing so, provide the American public with dedicated, competent and affordable health care.

From the standpoint of the medical profession itself, a self-regulated union would promote a standardization of medical care. It would ensure physician competence by establishing the guidelines for continuing medical education, obviate peer review organizations by sponsoring its own unbiased peer review activities and help put an end to the malpractice epidemic by operating efficient arbitration programs.

A medical union would also provide physicians with many badly needed services. It would standardize physicians' fees, create group purchasing networks, assist in physician placement, develop affordable malpractice and health insurance programs, provide a wide range of financial services, and create programs for rehabilitating impaired physicians, as well as career-modification programs for physicians who become disabled.

At a national level, such a union would allow the medical profession to create national health care policy rather than blindly follow it. It would allow the medical profession to elect physician-friendly legislators and put an end to the discriminatory treatment that the medical profession continues to receive at every level of government.

The creation of such a union would allow the medical profession to employ its own cadre of lawyers, researchers and public relations experts. It would allow the medical profession to start playing "hard ball," instead of "patty cake," with industry, the courts and our legislatures.

Closer to home, local chapters of a medical union would represent physicians in disputes with licensing boards, hospitals and third-party payers. They would work within the local communities to help guarantee smoke-free public facilities, drug-free schools and pollution-free environments, and help remove the hassle factor from medicine, thereby providing physicians more time for their professional activities.

During the next decade, the medical profession is going to find itself in an increasingly precarious position. With an unsteady economy, fewer and fewer patients are going to have health insurance.

With inadequate funding for medical research, the acquired immunodeficiency syndrome (AIDS), Alzheimer's and a number of other poorly understood diseases are going to have their own way with an ever-increasing number of patients. Society will invariably need somebody to blame for such a predictably deplorable state and, if history can be expected to repeat itself, the medical profession will be that somebody.

It can be argued the American Medical Association has attempted to unite American physicians in a medical union of sorts and has also attempted to protect the various interests of the medical profession. Unfortunately, the AMA has grown too complacent in its old age and has lost the ability to effectively fight for the rights of its members.

There may have been a day when the AMA was considered a perfect union but that day has long since passed. What the medical profession needs today is a more perfect union.

The American medical profession is arguably the world's greatest think tank and its members are arguably the world's most skilled professionals, but the profession's strength has been significantly diluted and its effectiveness significantly compromised by an inability to combine its abundant talents and energies. A more perfect union would effectively combine these abundant resources.

If the medical profession were to unionize, many of its current problems would find quick solutions and its remaining concerns would be no greater than America's historic need to find a good 5-cent cigar. If the medical profession fails to unionize in the near future, it may find itself stuck in a professional environment that has all the attributes of a 5-cent cigar – especially the smell.

October, 1992

THE STATELINESS OF MANAGED CARE

A lifelong resident of Long Island was transferred to a small southern town by his employer. Reluctantly, the man moved to the rural village where he immediately enrolled his son in the third grade of the community's only school.

Following the first day of school, the anxious father asked his son about his new educational experience.

"You know, Daddy," the boy replied enthusiastically, "I was the only student in my entire grade who could recite the multiplication tables."

"Well, that's because you're from Long Island," the proud father observed.

Following the boy's second day of school, the father once again inquired about his son's scholastic accomplishments.

"You know, Daddy," his son answered, "I was the only student in my grade who could name at least 10 American presidents."

"That's because you're from Long Island," the father remarked with obvious approval.

Following the third day of school, the father once again requested his daily progress report.

"You know, Daddy," the boy responded, "they gave us all physicals in school today, and the doctor told me I was one-foot taller than any other boy in my class. Is that because I'm from Long Island?"

"No, son," the father replied. "That's because you're 18!"

Many people have aversions about leaving home, and practically everyone can tell a story or two about unfortunate incidents that occurred while they were traveling out of state. Today, more than ever before, many of these stories concern difficulty receiving health care in another state because of health insurance restrictions.

For all intents and purposes, managed care patients have been forced to seek health care exclusively within their own managed care network. With few exceptions, such patients have encountered many obstacles when they have attempted to receive health care out of state, and an even greater number of obstacles when they have tried to have such health care services paid for by their managed care organizations.

Do the purveyors of managed care really expect people to stay home because of the possibility they may become ill or injured and require health care services? Do these managed care moguls really think it is fair to market managed care as a viable alternative to traditional health care when managed care will only pay for health care services obtained in a single network or in a single state?

The current managed care situation on both sides of the New York - Pennsylvania border is illustrative of the problems managed care patients encounter when they try to obtain health care services across state lines. To better understand a serious national problem that plagues many managed care patients who live near state borderlines, consider the following scenario.

If a patient, who is a member of a Northeastern Pennsylvania managed care network, sustains a life-threatening myocardial infarction in Great Bend, Pa., he cannot be taken by ambulance 15 minutes north to any of Binghamton, N.Y.'s three large teaching hospitals. Instead of being taken to hospitals that are amply staffed with cardiologists and cardiac surgeons, and equipped with state-of-the-art coronary care units and catheterization labs, the patient must be driven a comparable distance to a small Pennsylvania hospital that currently has 30 medical-surgical beds, 5 intensive care unit beds, no respirator, no Swan-Ganz capability and limited diagnostic equipment.

Patients who hold standard contracts with Northeastern Pennsylvania health maintenance organizations (HMOs) can, of course, bypass the managed care route and obtain medical services at a Binghamton hospital if they are willing to pay for their medical care out of pocket. Patients who hold "Point of Service" contracts with Northeastern Pennsylvania HMOs can also obtain medical care in Binghamton if they are willing to pay the difference between the actual cost of such care and the contribution of their HMO, which is currently 70% of the HMO's approved charges for services received, minus any deductibles.

In all honesty, the physicians who work at the previously-mentioned hospital in rural Pennsylvania are skilled, dedicated and capable of handling most medical emergencies, but complications do occur. Consequently, managed care patients with complicated myocardial infarctions that cannot be managed by these physicians at their small rural hospital must be transferred by ambulance 45 minutes south to the closest Pennsylvania referral hospital within the managed care network or a greater distance by helicopter to a larger intra-network teaching hospital.

When time is critical in the management of medical or surgical emergencies, does it make any sense to deny patients definitive care that is 15 minutes away just because a state line must be crossed and the patient's managed care organization is not licensed to operate across state lines? Does it make any sense to transport a patient with a life-threatening illness or injury 45 minutes by ambulance or helicopter to a hospital within a managed care network when the same definitive care could be obtained at any of a number of closer out of network or out of state hospitals in a matter of minutes?

If managed care is going to compete on the same playing field with traditional health care, it would seem managed care should be required by law to provide similar access to health care services. Insofar as managed care has already discovered how to find the money to pay the yearly $6 million compensation packages of many of its CEOs, it

181

would seem it should also be able to find the money to pay for timely and accessible emergency health care services for its members.

Managed care has many shortcomings, and limited access to medical and surgical care, especially when such care is obtained out of network and out of state, is one of the most serious. Not every third-grader knows how to recite the multiplication tables or name the presidents but, unlike many adults who are currently shaping managed care policy, most third-graders do know that a person who is having a heart attack should be taken to the closest hospital.

September, 1998

REVISITING *THE MALPRACTICE EPIDEMIC*

A few weeks ago, I received the following letter from a professional liability insurer:

"Dear Doctor, A short time ago, the Insurance Commissioner of Pennsylvania notified all professional liability insurance carriers of an anticipated shortfall in the Medical Professional Liability Loss Fund. The shortfall is estimated to range between $40 and $70 million for the calendar year running from 9/1/94 to 8/31/95. In case of insufficient funds, Section 701 (e)(3) of the Health Care Services Malpractice Act ("Act") authorizes the Pennsylvania Insurance Commissioner to levy an emergency surcharge on all health care providers during the month of September. The impact of the shortfall will likely require an emergency surcharge of approximately 20%-40% for all Pennsylvania health care providers.

"Please understand that an emergency surcharge has not been declared at this time. However, the purpose of this letter is to notify you of this potential and allow for financial preparation by you in the event contribution becomes necessary. If the commissioner does declare an emergency surcharge, notice will be given to us in September, 1995. Applicable Insurance Regulations require each carrier providing basic coverage to bill its insured health care providers the determined surcharge within fifteen (15) days after receipt of the Commissioner's notice. Payment becomes due within thirty (30) days of our notification to you. Failure to pay can result in disciplinary actions by the licensure board and/or loss of Fund coverage.

"Once again, this letter is to inform you of the anticipated emergency surcharge and allow you time to

183

financially prepare yourself. We will keep you informed as information becomes available....."

When *THE MALPRACTICE EPIDEMIC* was first published in 1990, many readers were shocked to discover U.S. courts were handing out nearly $30 billion a year in malpractice settlements. Other readers were shocked to learn diagnostic tests, consultations and other defensive medicine practices that were employed by physicians to protect themselves against malpractice suits were costing American health care consumers another $30 billion yearly.

Still other readers were shocked to discover that, on a national level, victorious plaintiffs in malpractice suits were only taking home 28% of the money they were awarded in court. The lawyers, as well as expert witnesses and others employed by the lawyers to help win their cases, were taking home the rest.

When I wrote *THE MALPRACTICE EPIDEMIC*, I attempted to expose the unscrupulous activity of the American legal profession, the profiteering of the American insurance industry and the collusion of these two groups with the body politic. It was my hope the book would open a few eyes and ultimately set the stage for true and lasting health care reform.

A lot has happened since 1990. For starters, managed care has forced physicians to cut corners with their patients so insurance companies could continue to post strong corporate earnings and their CEO's could continue to collect yearly multi-million-dollar performance bonuses.

Medicare has continued to force physicians to treat patients using diagnosis-related groups (DRGs), and the hospital days thereunto pertaining, rather than scientific acumen, compassion and common sense. Using phony audits, biased peer review and consumer-directed propaganda, Medicare, like managed care, has forced physicians to practice medicine while wearing handcuffs.

The creation of a national malpractice data bank has made it more difficult for malpractice suits to be settled quietly and amicably out of court. To avoid listing in the federal registry, physicians have been forced to settle malpractice suits in courtrooms where the monetary settlements far exceed those made out of court.

Finally, our state and federal governments have taken sides with the legal profession and insurance industry, and have joined in the fight to gain total and absolute control over the American medical profession. Lawyers have been allowed to file simultaneous civil and criminal suits in alleged acts of medical malpractice, courts have granted exorbitant malpractice awards that have forced physicians into personal bankruptcy and insurance companies have been allowed to continually increase malpractice insurance premiums without justification.

All the while, the judicial branch of government has sanctified the greed of the American legal profession, and the legislative branch of government has enacted laws that continue to support the interests of big business and thwart those of the medical profession. Under the guise of health care reform, politicians have protected the special interests of business and the law, blamed the current health care mess on the incompetence, avarice and unfeeling nature of the American medical profession, and effectively alienated many Americans from their physicians.

The end result has been a perpetuation of the malpractice epidemic. The end result has also been the insidious development of a milieu that allows physicians to render competent, and often heroic, medical care for the right to lose their fortunes in a court of law, the right to be treated like criminals and the right to pay surcharges so the shortfalls of professional liability loss funds might be offset.

The medical literature has recently been filled with reports of impending physician oversupply in the United States, but none of these reports have considered the effect of malpractice litigation on current and future membership in the American medical profession. The malpractice

185

epidemic has already caused too many physicians to prematurely leave the medical profession, and it has caused too many of the remaining physicians to practice medicine without spirit, interest or many of the other attributes that lend purpose and meaning to their work.

A number of medical economists have postulated the year 2000 may witness a statistical oversupply of physicians in the United States. Without timely malpractice reform, however, a significant percentage of these physicians promise to be little more than shadows of the physicians a wiser, kinder and more appreciative society might have allowed.

Our nation's current health care crisis is and always has been directly related to the malpractice epidemic. When our nation finally learns how to identify acts of medical malpractice in a just fashion and compensate the victims of medical malpractice in an equitable manner, America will have taken a giant step toward achieving health care reform.

In the meantime, I've got to figure out a way to come up with some bucks for this surcharge. Maybe it's time to publish another book!

November, 1995

MALPRACTICE CRISIS IN PENNSYLVANIA

This past February, I received a letter from my malpractice insurer informing me Pennsylvania House Bill 44 had passed and, as a result, I qualified for some malpractice insurance relief in the form of a partial or complete abatement of my Mcare assessments for 2003 and 2004. Mcare stands for the "Medical Care Availability and Reduction of Error Fund," a fund controlled by the Pennsylvania Insurance Department.

The Mcare assessment is that portion of a physician's malpractice premium that is applied to the "Pennsylvania Medical Professional Liability Catastrophe Loss Fund." This fund pays malpractice awards in excess of the physician's insurance policy limits, or awards in excess of monies paid by the physician's malpractice insurer to settle a claim.

The legislation was passed in response to the exodus of many physicians from Pennsylvania due, in part, to many years of skyrocketing malpractice premiums and an unfavorable malpractice climate. The malpractice crisis started to escalate in Pennsylvania a decade ago when physicians were forced to pay additional surcharges to help refuel a nearly depleted Catastrophe Loss Fund.

Partial or complete Mcare assessment relief for a limited period of time was Pennsylvania's attempt at retaining its physicians. Unfortunately, the gesture was too little and too late to retain the many specialists who had already left Pennsylvania because they could no longer afford the exorbitant malpractice insurance premiums that would allow them to continue practicing in the state.

To receive Mcare abatements for 2003 and/or 2004, Pennsylvania physicians were required to file applications to Pennsylvania's "Health Care Provider Retention

Program." Separate applications had to be filed for each year the physicians were requesting abatements.

The applications required personal, specialty, practice and insurance information from physicians, as well as answers to questions concerning any adverse events in the physicians' practices. The applications also required physicians to sign retention pledges to continue practicing medicine in Pennsylvania.

To be eligible for an abatement of the 2003 Mcare assessment, physicians had to agree to continue practicing medicine in Pennsylvania until December 31, 2004. To be eligible for the 2004 abatement, physicians had to agree to practice until December 31, 2005.

The "Certificate Of Retention Pledge To Practice" for 2004 reads as follows:

"I hereby attest that I have applied for an abatement of my 2004 Mcare assessment, which may include a request for refund or credit for the amount of 2004 Mcare assessment that I paid and, which may have been remitted by my primary carrier to Mcare, before enactment of the Health Care Provider Retention Program ("Program"). I agree to continue to provide health care services in the Commonwealth of Pennsylvania through December 31, 2005, pursuant to the Program.

"If I cease providing health care services in the Commonwealth of Pennsylvania prior to December 31, 2005, I will be in violation of the required terms and conditions of the Program, and I will be required to repay Mcare the abated amount in full, plus administrative and legal costs, if applicable.

"Any amount owed to the Commonwealth of Pennsylvania as a result of the cessation of provision of health care services referenced above and the repayment obligation of any abated amount owed is considered a tax obligation, and is subject to collection efforts and any other penalties provided by law associated with non-payment of a tax obligation to the Commonwealth of Pennsylvania."

Having practiced medicine in rural Northeastern Pennsylvania since 1981, and not planning any out of state moves in the foreseeable future, I applied for 2003 and 2004 Mcare abatements this past February and pledged to continue practicing in Pennsylvania. In March, I received notification I was eligible for a 50% 2003 Mcare abatement, and I should expect to receive a refund "at least 3 months" from the date of my eligibility notice.

To date, 4 months later, I still have not received my 2003 Mcare refund. I have, however, received separate notification that I am also eligible for a 50% 2004 Mcare abatement, and had that abatement credited by my insurer to the recent malpractice insurance bill I received a few days following notification of my 2004 eligibility.

In that bill, I was credited $2,623 for my 2004 50% Mcare abatement. In that same bill, the insurer raised my premium $1,432, even though my malpractice record is clean.

My savings by agreeing to participate in the 2004 Pennsylvania "Health Care Provider Retention Program" – pocket change. My savings by agreeing to participate in the 2003 program – pocket change, said to be in the mail.

The cost of learning why Pennsylvania still has a malpractice crisis on its hands - priceless! Well, in my case, 50% of priceless!

July, 2004

KNOWING WHAT TO KNOW

Not that many moons ago, physicians administered oxygen in a manner that would be considered unsophisticated by today's standards. Premature infants, for example, were routinely given 100% oxygen without regard to arterial oxygen concentrations.

One of the developments that ended this practice and forced the medical profession to devise more precise ways to administer oxygen was the discovery of the relationship between oxygen administration and retrolental fibroplasia. In this condition, also known as Terry's Syndrome, opaque tissue forms behind the lens, gradually resulting in retinal detachment, an arrest of normal eye growth and blindness.

For many years, many competent physicians administered high concentrations of oxygen to premature infants, unaware that oxygen so administered could lead to retrolental fibroplasia. When the association between this ophthalmic disorder and oxygen therapy was finally established, many of these physicians were sued for malpractice.

In court, defense attorneys argued the physicians who administered 100% oxygen to preemies were not guilty of malpractice because the medical profession was unaware of the deleterious effects of administering oxygen in high concentrations. The plaintiffs' attorneys disagreed.

During the same era when it was still considered standard medical practice to give 100% oxygen to premature infants, an article appeared in a foreign medical journal. This article detailed the development of retrolental fibroplasia in lab animals that had been given oxygen in concentrations greater than 40%.

The plaintiffs' attorneys argued that an apparent link between the administration of oxygen in high concentrations and the insidious development of retrolental fibroplasia had been reported in the scientific literature, and physicians who continued to give 100% oxygen to premature infants following the publication of this report were negligent. The argument stood up in court and those afflicted with Terry's Syndrome won their cases.

Very few of the physicians who were successfully sued for malpractice ever heard of the foreign medical journal in which the report had been published; none of the physicians had ever read the report. Still, the court ruled it was a physician's responsibility to keep abreast of scientific developments that could affect patient care - even developments that were reported in journals not commonly read by most physicians.

Today, with computers, television and the information superhighway, medical information is more accessible than it was a half-century ago. For that matter, this information is more accessible than it was a decade ago.

Still, medical information continues to exist outside the mainstream - typically in periodicals that are not widely read or listed in medical references, such as *Index Medicus*. As a consequence, physicians continue to labor without information they may one day be expected to know.

To test this point, I recently polled a number of primary care physicians who administer allergen-specific immunotherapy or "allergy shots" in their offices. These physicians were asked to list the emergency resuscitation equipment and medications in their office that could be used to treat an anaphylactic reaction to an allergy shot; they were also asked to name or describe any references that specifically recommended which equipment and medications a medical office should have before allergy shots were administered.

Most of the physicians polled stated they routinely kept epinephrine and some kind of intramuscular steroid preparation in their offices but very few had immediate access to intravenous hydrocortisone or any of the intravenous drugs commonly used during advanced cardiac life support. All of the physicians had electrocardiogram machines in their offices but very few had cardiac monitors, defibrillators, endotracheal intubation equipment, manual resuscitators, portable oxygen or sterile intravenous fluids.

None of the physicians polled could remember ever reading a journal article or medical textbook chapter devoted to the emergency equipment and medications that should be present in a medical office before allergy shots were administered. All of the physicians polled acknowledged that anaphylactic shock and cardio-pulmonary collapse could follow the administration of allergen-specific immunotherapy but the majority of the physicians felt such life-threatening sequellae were so rare that medical offices did not have to be equipped with emergency resuscitation equipment and drugs as a prerequisite to administering allergy shots.

A few years ago, an allergist published a paper in the quarterly review of a teaching hospital. The paper listed the emergency resuscitation equipment and drugs that have been previously mentioned as items that should be present in a medical office before allergy shots were administered.

In doing so, the allergist presented his personal opinion rather than a recommendation based on exhaustive experience or research. Such a written opinion, however, would be more ammunition than most malpractice lawyers needed to destroy a physician whose poorly-equipped office was the site of a maloccurrence that followed the administration of an allergy shot.

There are physicians whose offices are adequately equipped to handle life-threatening emergencies. There are also physicians who have been unable to justify the expense of equipping a medical office with emergency resuscitation gear and supplies that might never be used.

Whether or not a physician needs emergency resuscitation equipment and supplies on hand before allergy shots are given is unclear. What is much clearer is the predictable reaction of the courts and news media to physicians who are found negligent following therapeutic maloccurrences.

To this end, state and national licensing boards, as well as medical societies, need to become more involved in the process of developing specific, clear-cut guidelines for the practice of medicine. Where controversial issues concerning emergency equipment and protocols exist, such boards and societies need to issue official statements that will clearly define the nature and scope of accepted medical practice.

These licensing boards and medical societies should also review the medical literature, including esoteric periodicals, for articles and reports that might impact on the practice of medicine. Thought-provoking articles and reports should be brought to the attention of the physicians governed by these boards and societies, while frivolous articles that could be misconstrued to the detriment of physicians should be publicly refuted by these same groups.

Care must be given by licensing boards and medical societies to keep their research intellectually honest at all times. Political pressure and the unscrupulous efforts of self-serving industries that stand to profit by the manner in which physicians practice medicine must by recognized and excluded from the dissemination of the unbiased findings and conclusions of the licensing boards and medical societies.

There was a time when such widespread literature reviews would have been impractical. Today, however, the internet has made these reviews practical just as the malpractice epidemic has made them necessary.

Science has been previously defined as a unified body of knowledge. This being the case, it would appear the time has come for medicine to become more scientific in its approach to taking care of business.

Physicians need to become more unified in the way medicine is practiced, offices are equipped and information is disseminated. Physicians can start doing this for themselves or continue to watch as it is done for them by the courts, legislatures, and industries that sponsor self-serving research and generate spurious research findings.

There is a tremendous amount of information physicians need to know. The mission of every physician would be greatly facilitated by knowing what to know.

September, 1996

SENSES AND SENSIBILITY

Recently, I had the honor of speaking at the annual conference of one of our country's oldest and most prestigious medical societies. The topic of my speech was managed care.

Realizing I would be speaking to hundreds of highly respected physicians on a topic of monumental importance, I spent a great deal of time preparing a speech that would convincingly portray the reality of the topic at hand. For a few months, I reviewed volumes of material and carefully composed a speech that would fit into the one hour that had been allotted to my presentation.

When I arrived at the site of the conference, I was informed by the society's executive director that a large health maintenance organization (HMO) was protesting my appearance. Through its medical director, the HMO complained that the society should not feature any speaker who might have anything unfavorable to say about managed care.

When the society's executive director reminded the HMO spokesman that representatives of various HMOs were given the opportunity to speak at previous conferences sponsored by the medical society, the HMO director continued to protest. He argued his HMO's catchment area was underpenetrated by managed care and physicians who still hadn't joined managed care should not be listening to one of managed care's most vocal opponents.

Before all was said and done, the medical society's executive director, physician conference director and president were contacted by the medical director of the HMO, as were various physicians who were attending the conference. Fortunately, those who invited me to speak remembered why they invited me, and my speech was

197

delivered as scheduled to the overwhelming satisfaction of a large audience.

Immediately following my speech, I offered to meet with any and all HMO representatives to publicly debate the issue of managed care. As might be expected, no one accepted my invitation.

A few weeks after the conference, I received a letter from the medical society's executive director. "After carefully reviewing the evaluation forms," the director wrote, "it appears that most physicians must have agreed with you because you received all 4's and 5's with 5 being our highest rating."

Most physicians and most patients will agree with the truth when the truth is presented to them. Unfortunately, managed care has been inconsistent in its ability to present the truth to health care consumers and providers.

If managed care is on the up-and-up, why won't HMOs share their secrets with doctors and patients? Are the HMOs afraid someone will finally discover the managed care equation has health care rationing to patients plus payment rationing to physicians equaling excessive profits for the health maintenance corporations?

Newsweek recently polled 150 of America's largest HMOs to formulate a national HMO ranking. Only 88 HMOs provided the publication with sufficient information to permit such an exercise.

If managed care is on the square, what does it have to hide? Why are HMOs so afraid of making the truth public?

Before the Second Continental Congress entertained the concept of American independence from England, a motion for debate on the question of independence had to be passed. With the vote for debate deadlocked, the final vote was given to an elderly Rhode Island rum guzzler by the name of Stephen Hopkins.

Stating he had never "seen, heard nor smelled" any issue that couldn't be discussed, Hopkins voted to debate the question of American independence. His vote helped set the stage for the birth of the United States of America.

Unlike Hopkins, too many of those who are paid to speak on behalf of America's HMOs, have never seen, heard nor smelled any managed care issue they feel comfortable discussing in public or allowing anyone outside the managed care arena to discuss. What they have seen is the hostile takeover of a one-trillion-dollar health care industry by their corporations, what they have heard are the rumors government officials are behind the takeover and what they have smelled is the resulting decay of health care in America.

March, 1998

GOVERNMENT SPENDING CUTS

Nestled in Pennsylvania's beautiful Pocono Mountains is the tiny hamlet of Tobyhanna. In addition to a state park and a few taverns, the town is best known as the home of the Tobyhanna Army Depot.

My father was one of the depot's first employees. Starting as a safety officer and then becoming the depot's Safety Director, he spent the better part of twenty years working at Tobyhanna.

Most of my father's professional life was spent in government service. Following World War II and a long tour of duty as an infantry sergeant in the Philippines, he worked for the Veteran's Administration before transferring to Tobyhanna.

With the promise of an early retirement, he left Tobyhanna after two decades of service and spent the last few years of his professional life developing a safety office for the Federal Communications Commission in Washington, D.C. He retired at age 55, and one year to the day of his retirement, he sustained a myocardial infarction and died en route to a hospital.

My father died on the first day of my senior year at Temple Med. His unexpected death made for a less-than-auspicious start to my final year in medical school.

My father enjoyed each of his jobs, but working at Tobyhanna was something special. He took pride in the fact he was one of the depot's pioneers, one of the major reasons for the depot's exemplary safety records and one of the first to envision the facility's enormous potential.

For the past few months, the Tobyhanna Army Depot has been in the news. In an age of unprecedented government spending cuts, the depot is one of the military installations currently being threatened with closure.

It is no secret our country has a problem with a rapidly growing federal deficit. Accordingly, politicians are in the process of trying to erase the deficit by dramatically retrenching in the areas of defense, human services and health care.

Unfortunately, by taking the axe to many existing federally-funded programs, our political leaders are making the mistake of being penny-wise and pound-foolish. They are trying to take control of the federal deficit but, in doing so, they are creating problems beyond their wildest imagination.

For example, by closing the Tobyhanna Army Depot, the federal government will be taking jobs away from thousands of Northeastern Pennsylvania residents who, by the way, also pay federal and state income tax. Northeastern Pennsylvania doesn't have a few thousand extra jobs to hand out to the people who are currently employed at Tobyhanna.

Consequently, closing the Tobyhanna Army Depot will add many names to the unemployment rolls and, with time, many of these same names will be transferred to the welfare and disability rolls. Federal and state taxes will eventually be used to sustain many individuals who are now gainfully employed at Tobyhanna but, unlike the current scenario, the federal and state governments will no longer profit from the work being done at Tobyhanna and will have nothing to show for the money they dole out in unemployment, welfare and disability payments.

Finally, closing the Tobyhanna Army Depot will significantly harm the economy of the geographic area that surrounds the depot, as well as the economy of the various towns Tobyhanna employees currently call home. Every time another military base like Tobyhanna is closed in the United States, someone's economy suffers but, more importantly, people suffer.

Just as the federal government is attempting to cut defense spending by placing military installations on the chopping block, it is also attempting to cut spending by reducing the manpower in our armed forces. The thinking is any future military confrontations that involve the United States will be handled by Stealth Bombers, Smart Missiles and, if all else fails, "The Big One."

What our politicians fail to realize, however, is armed forces may one day be required to ensure peace and domestic tranquility within the borders of the United States. Our nation is home to an ever-increasing number of armed militias, terrorist groups and subversives who, at any given moment, could easily create the kind of havoc we recently witnessed in Oklahoma City.

If any insurrection were to occur within the borders of the United States, dropping an atomic bomb would not be a plausible military option. A more realistic option would be military troops - and lots of them.

Our federal government has spent the better part of a century, untold lives and incomprehensible amounts of tax-payers' money creating a strong national defense. To thoughtlessly dismantle our defense and leave our nation vulnerable to foreign or domestic attack is the mark of a government that has lost its ability to establish priorities, provide for the unexpected and, in essence, think critically.

Just as the federal government is showing thoughtless disregard for our defense needs, it is currently showing the same kind of fuzzy thinking by suggesting further cuts in health and human services spending. High on the list of such spending cuts are the Medicare and Medicaid programs.

Medicare was created by the federal government to provide health care to the elderly and disabled. Medicaid was created to provide health care to the indigent.

Every time the federal government tampers with the Medicare or Medicaid programs, the disenchanted and "poor but proud" in our midst cut back on their utilization of health care services. When this happens, preventive medicine gives way to emergency medical services, hospitalizations and skilled nursing care, and the cost of caring for the elderly, disabled and indigent, who would rather forego timely medical intervention than pay higher co-payments and deductibles or allow themselves to be considered charity cases, dramatically increases.

Every time the government tampers with Medicare or Medicaid, emergency rooms across the country experience dramatically increased utilization and hospitals experience dramatically increased financial losses. Where the government saves in one area, the nation loses in another.

The government's typical response to such a problem is to create a new task force and initiate an expensive government review that invariably results in the creation of new government programs. To paraphrase Alabama's illustrious Gump family, "Bureaucracy is as bureaucracy does."

Speaking for myself, I don't want any more cuts in defense spending. Actually, I would like to see more defense spending.

I would like to be able to go to sleep at night knowing the United States is adequately protected against foreign and domestic enemies. I would also like to see our government providing more Americans with employment opportunities in the armed forces and in military support facilities like the Tobyhanna Army Depot.

I don't mind paying my fair share of taxes. If I had my druthers, though, I'd rather be paying taxes for tangible services than unemployment, welfare and disability programs.

Just as I don't want any more cuts in defense spending, I also don't want any more cuts in the health and human services sector. Once again, I would like to see more government spending in these areas for reasons so apparent as to obviate explanation.

So, how are we, as Americans, to pay for more defense, more health care for our elderly and indigent and more human services for our needy? How are we, as a nation, to maintain the status of our quo without raising the taxes of the average working man and woman and, at the same time, control our federal deficit?

For starters, we need to stop building billion-dollar facilities and million-dollar toys that we ultimately give away to other nations or slick entrepreneurs for pennies on the dollar. Next, we need to stop our profligate spending by taking a close look at how much we are paying for goods and services to the United States government.

In the health care arena, we need to simplify payment for services to Medicare and Medicaid beneficiaries. This will allow us to eliminate many of the Medicare and Medicaid audit and research programs and, in the process, save untold millions of dollars annually.

Finally, we need to reform our methods of taxation. We need to adopt new and more effective methods of having each American pay his or her fair share of tax.

There are physicians, defense experts and businessmen in this country who could sit down with representatives of the appropriate government agencies and identify and correct the pressing problems of those agencies in an expeditious manner. Unfortunately, such efficiency experts are not a part of our government's bureaucracy - and we all know what the Gumps might say about that.

We need to open the doors of government to real experts who can teach government how to operate more efficiently. We need to open the doors of government to America.

Plans to close the Tobyhanna Army Depot and carelessly decimate other federal facilities, programs and jobs clearly demonstrate the shortsightedness of contemporary American government. Millions of Americans spent their entire professional lives in government-sponsored activities, and many of these activities are now being thoughtlessly abandoned without regard to the potential consequences.

A nation can only be as great as its people and, to be great, people must have the chance to be productive. I learned that a long time ago from the Safety Director of the Tobyhanna Army Depot.

June, 1995

MY DREAM DATE WITH HILLARY

I had another one of those crazy dreams again last night.

I was home alone, trying to memorize the 64000 series of Medicare billing codes, when I heard the front doorbell ring. When I opened the door, I couldn't believe my eyes.

"Hi, Bernie," she said, diplomatically offering me her hand. "I'm Hillary."

"I know who you are," I said. "Please come in."

"Are you alone," she asked, as she tucked a monogrammed leather attaché case under her arm.

"Well, I guess no one is ever really alone," I replied.

"Oh, an existential/phenomenologist," she said with a smile. "I like that in a man."

Escorting Hillary into the blue room, I left her admiring a paint-by-the-numbers mural while I went searching for some liquid refreshment. When I returned, she was looking at herself in the reflections of my white baby grand piano and toying with her hair.

"A new do?" I asked, as I handed her a drink.

"Much ado about nothing," she replied lightly.

"Shakespeare," I observed. "I like that in a woman."

As Hillary sat down with her bottle of YooHoo, I looked straight into her eyes and slugged down a shot of 114-proof bourbon. As steam escaped from my ears and bonding material started to melt in one of my upper molars, I maintained eye contact with Hillary and quickly downed a large schooner of brewski.

Hillary sighed nervously and fumbled with her soda straw. Just then, I eased over to the piano and started playing, "In the Mood."

"You're angry, aren't you?" she observed.

"How can you tell?" I asked. "Is it the way I handle my liquor?"

"No, it's the way you're playing, "In The Mood," she replied. "I've never heard it played with an augmented C7 before."

"It's the only song I know how to play on the piano," I answered.

"That explains it," she said. "I guess I've just gotten used to the way my husband plays the song on his saxophone."

"I used to play the saxophone I grade school," I offered enthusiastically, "but I finally gave it up after learning only one song."

"What song was that," she asked inquisitively.

"In The Mood," I replied.

As Hillary took another short sip of YooHoo and started talking to me with her eyes, I felt as though I could tell her anything.

"Hillary, I am angry," I admitted, as I sat down beside her. "I'm angry because of this smoke screen everyone's calling a health care task force. I'm angry because millions of Americans are counting on health care reform they won't be getting anytime soon. I'm angry because the kids aren't going to get the vaccines they were promised, the poor aren't going to get the health insurance they were promised and the patients aren't going to get the cures they were promised."

Hillary just stared at me.

"And you know what else?" I asked. "I'm angry because managed care is going to make medicine more of a business than it already is. And I'm angry because my destiny as a physician is going to be determined by the lobbyists who come up with the biggest political action contributions. And I'm angry because all of this could have been prevented."

Hillary continued to stare.

"Don't you see?" I asked, watching Hillary nervously shrink into a corner of the couch. "The problems of two small people don't amount to a hill of beans in this crazy world, but the problems of 200 million people amount to a lot of beans. This country needs health care reform, but we'll never have it as long as a bunch of amateurs keep trying to resurrect a system that's too broke to fix."

"I've never heard it put quite like that before," Hillary responded.

"Ditto," I replied.

As Hillary continued to stare at me, it started to become obvious that she knew that I knew.

"I wish I could stay longer," she said nervously, as she started to get up from the couch, "but it's late and I must be going."

With one final loud slurp, Hillary finished her YooHoo before heading toward the foyer.

"This night will always be special to me," she said, with an extra measure of sincerity.

Following one last look into each other's eyes, Hillary smiled again and quietly left. As she faded into the darkness, only the sound of her whistling, In The Mood, broke the stillness of the night.

Just as I began to savor my dream, my sleep was interrupted by the shrill ringing of the telephone.

"C'mon, Doc, shake it out. It's almost 6 A.M.," Babs Gordon, the eighty-year-old president of the local Gray Panthers chapter shouted over the phone. "What you plannin' on doin'? Sleepin' in till the crack of noon?"

"What's the problem, Babs?" I asked in a stuporous tone of voice.

"Well, me and the Panthers had a meetin' last night," she answered, "and we all came to the conclusion that you should get in touch with Hillary and send her and that blue-ribbon task force of hers some of your ideas on health care reform."

"Why?" I asked.

"Ain't you never heard of the HCFA?" Babs asked.

"You mean the Health Care Financing Administration?" I inquired.

"Not anymore," Babs replied. "Now it stands for 'Hillary Can Fix Anything.'"

"Babs," I asked, "what would you say if I told you Hillary came to my house last night to discuss health care reform?"

"I'd say, 'In your dreams, Cowboy,'" Babs answered, as she hung up the phone.

"In my dreams," I thought, as I climbed out of bed with a strange craving for a bottle of YooHoo. I guess health care reform has to start somewhere.

August, 1993

ABOUT THE AUTHOR

BERNARD LEO REMAKUS, M.D. is a native of Wilkes-Barre, Pa. He received his B.S. degree from King's College, M.Ed. degree from East Stroudsburg State College, and M.D. degree from the Temple University School of Medicine. He completed a three-year residency in internal medicine at Abington Memorial Hospital which led to his certification as a Diplomate of the American Board of Internal Medicine.

Dr. Remakus has practiced internal medicine in a rural, physician-shortage area of Northeastern Pennsylvania for 40 years. During that time, he has published five novels – *The Paraclete, Keystone, Cassidy's Solution, Mia* and *The Lame Duck*; three works of non-fiction – *The Malpractice Epidemic, Medicine From The Heart* and *Medicine Between The Lines*; and one screenplay, *Mia*.

He has also authored more than 200 scientific articles that have been published in: *The New England Journal of Medicine, the Journal of the American Medical Association, Newsweek, Medical Economics, The Archives of Internal Medicine, Internal Medicine News, Consultant, Geriatrics, Modern Medicine, Medical World News, Hospital News, The American Magazine, Pride, KevinMD,* and *Internal Medicine World Report*. Many of these articles have been reprinted in popular newspapers and magazines.

From 1991 to 2002, Dr. Remakus was the featured columnist and a member of the Editorial Advisory Board of the medical publication, *Internal Medicine World Report*. His column in that publication had the distinction of being one of the most widely read and longest running physician-written columns in America.

When not practicing medicine or writing, Dr. Remakus serves as a professional speaker and Clinical Assistant Professor at the Temple University School of

Medicine. In previous years, he has also performed clinical drug research, worked as a medical examiner and consultant, and coached his local high school baseball team to a league championship and four post-season district playoff appearances in six seasons.

The recipient of numerous awards and citations, Dr. Remakus received the *Albert Nelson Marquis Lifetime Achievement Award* in 2020. He is listed in *Who's Who in America, Who's Who in The World, Who's Who in Medicine and Healthcare, Who's Who in Science and Engineering,* and *Who's Who in American Education.*

Dr. Remakus and his wife, Charlotte, have been married for 46 years, and their three children, Chris, Ali and Matt, are all physicians. Their son-in-law, Mark, is also a physician, and their daughter-in-law, Sanda, is a Ph.D. in medical microbiology. Dr. and Mrs. Remakus have four grandchildren, Jake, Betsy, Anabelle and Charlie.

www.ingramcontent.com/pod-product-compliance
Lightning Source LLC
Chambersburg PA
CBHW051802170526
45167CB00005B/1847